Improving Cognitive Function After Cancer

Shelli Kesler, PhD

ISBN-13: 978-1490367729

ISBN-10: 1490367721

Table of Contents

Introduction

I began putting together this guide several years ago when I started seeing more and more patients with cancer in my clinical neuropsychology practice. I found it very useful to provide patients with a written reference of the information we discussed in treatment sessions.   As my clinical and research interests moved entirely to cancer-related cognitive difficulties, I was able to greatly expand this guide with evidence-based information from work by my own laboratory as well as that of my colleagues in this field.

This book was written specifically for cancer survivors who are struggling with cognitive side effects following cancer and/or cancer treatments.   However, practitioners, family members and friends who care for these survivors might also find it useful.   Chapters 1 through 3 discuss some of the candidate mechanisms underlying cancer-related cognitive difficulties and describe some of the symptoms of these difficulties. Chapters 5 through 9 provide suggestions and guidelines for coping with cognitive effects including specific strategies for improving memory, thinking and attention.

However, this guide should not be considered a substitute for medical care. Chapter 4 provides information regarding the type of clinical care that patients should consider in order to address cognitive difficulties that are interfering with their daily functioning.

I organized the book with individuals who might have cognitive difficulties in mind.   Therefore, important information is repeated and summarized. Less familiar terms are defined in the text where possible and again in the glossary. Glossary terms appear in bold font. Illustrations are provided to aid in understanding and learning.

In some sections of this book, I provide examples of commercially available products or services. These examples are based on my own experiences and preferences. This does not mean that I have done extensive comparative research regarding all available products. There are many other options that readers might select instead. Also, it should be noted that I do not receive any financial or other incentives for my suggestions.

People often ask me if I would undergo chemotherapy treatment should I be diagnosed with cancer and my answer is yes. There are many difficult side effects to chemotherapy and other cancer treatments. Cognitive dysfunction is just one of several issues that cancer survivors might face. However, adjuvant treatments like chemotherapy have profoundly improved survival rates. Our understanding of treatment side effects, including cognitive difficulties, has exponentially increased during the past decade. While there are many questions that remain, efforts to answer them are ongoing.

For example, there is an international group of researchers dedicated to this issue – the International Cognition and Cancer Task Force (http://www.icctf.com). The National Cancer Institute, National Institute of Nursing Research and others have made research in this area a priority with increased funding opportunities and initiatives. Cognitive effects of cancer and its treatments have received tremendous attention from the media and press during the past several years, vastly increasing public and professional awareness. I have great hope that continued research will lead to increasingly effective interventions for treating and perhaps even preventing cognitive dysfunction associated with cancer and its treatments.

Forward

Improving Cognitive Function After Cancer is an essential book with invaluable information and proactive solutions for everyone who faces challenges in cognitive functioning after cancer. I previously worked as a mechanical engineer and computer engineer in very demanding and challenging positions. In 2006, I was diagnosed with breast cancer. After treatment, I could not function cognitively at the same level as before cancer and I struggled significantly to perform at work. When I tried to talk to my oncologists about this, they told me that cancer treatment could not be the cause. I was eventually let go from my job and later denied disability because no one understood or would acknowledge the problem of chemo brain. I felt extremely frustrated and invalidated. I knew then that I would have to find someone with the answers on my own.

During my searching, I found Dr. Kesler at Stanford. I liked her approach to addressing chemo brain and I believed her strategies would be most helpful to me so I traveled from Florida to California. I had many questions such as, why could I not keep track of what I was doing? Why was it so difficult for me to think of how to start a project or what steps to do next? Why was I often so confused when talking with certain people? Dr. Kesler had answers. I was very excited to finally have some explanations for my experiences and some help in addressing my cognitive challenges.

Dr. Kesler designed a cognitive rehabilitation program for me. She equipped me with principles, techniques and strategies that I could utilize to improve my successes. These proactive solutions are empowering to me. She has now written this powerful book to help people like me. This book contains her approach to the challenges and issues that I faced. I have experienced tremendous improvements and successes. My flexibility in thinking and my problem solving have improved. I am better able to communicate with others, especially physicians. My working memory has improved. I am better able to hold more information in my head and work with it. My ability to drive has improved because now I am able to keep track of the constantly changing environment, anticipate, plan and execute efficiently. I am faster and more efficient at performing tasks. I am able to function at a higher level with more confidence.

Dr. Kesler presents a well-designed "plan of action" that uses multifaceted strategies that can synergistically provide optimal results. Her book is well researched, evidence-based and written in a logical and easy flowing manner. She describes the "whys" with thoughtful reasoning so you will be able to gain a deeper understanding of why the interventions work independently but also more powerfully when the strategies are combined.   Dr. Kesler is an accomplished researcher with expertise in chemo brain. She is a pioneer in chemo brain research and has demonstrated that it is real; why it is real and how it impairs cognitive functioning. I believe she is a true innovator in translating her research into creative workable solutions for patients. It is also evident to me that she is passionate about her work and she also has compassion for her patients and sincerely wants to make a difference for cancer survivors. Dr. Kesler has been a life saver for me and instrumental in my substantial neurological and cognitive improvements. She has given me tremendous support and encouragement through this journey. She gave me hope that I can overcome the barriers and challenges that I have encountered with chemo brain.

I highly recommend this book to all patients and families who are experiencing the challenges and frustrations of chemo brain. I sincerely believe the answers, interventions, and techniques provided by Dr. Kesler can provide a positive impact and return of hope. The content of this book will also be of great benefit to healthcare providers everywhere to help in understanding the realities and challenges of chemo brain that their patients face. It is my sincere hope and plea that they will take the information in these pages and use it and then take the time to listen and acknowledge the symptoms and challenges of their cancer patients with chemo brain. Dismissing the complaints as invalid or imaginary only adds to the problems and issues. However, the healthcare provider can be a part of the solution by offering support and understanding by pointing out to the patient that there are answers as well as possible interventions.

Linda Dance, M.E., P.E.

Software Engineer, Breast Cancer Survivor

Chapter 1: Cancer and Cognition

Cognitive difficulties such as problems with thinking, **memory** and **attention**, are a common complication following cancer and cancer treatments. When considering the effects of central nervous system (**CNS**) cancer, such as brain tumor or brain metastases, this may seem unsurprising. However, a large percentage of patients with non-CNS cancers such as breast, prostate and lung cancers as well as leukemia and lymphoma also experience cognitive changes [1]. Patients who have received chemotherapy are 3-5 times more likely to have cognitive difficulties compared to those who have not received chemotherapy [2,3]. As a result, cognitive problems following cancer are often referred to as "**chemo brain**".

However, patients who are treated with radiation to the head and/or neck are also at higher risk for having cognitive difficulties. Hematopoietic stem cell transplant has been associated with cognitive dysfunction [1]. Patients who have received local radiation and/or hormonal blockade medications without chemotherapy can demonstrate cognitive difficulties [4]. Even patients with non-CNS cancer who have not yet started adjuvant therapies can show altered cognitive function [5,6].

A growing body of research suggests that cognitive difficulties in patients with cancer stem from brain changes that occur following cancer and/or cancer treatments. In patients with brain tumor, these brain changes are often obvious. There tends to be tissue damage in the regions surrounding the tumor site. However, tumors are also associated with shifting of brain tissue that can result in less obvious damage to regions distant from the tumor. Brain tumors also cause **white matter** alteration including disruption, displacement and infiltration of white matter pathways [7,8]. White matter is important for connecting specialized brain regions together and facilitating communication within and between **brain networks**. Thus, a brain tumor could result in disruption of multiple brain systems and impairment in a variety of cognitive functions.

Some patients with leukemia or lymphoma receive intrathecal chemotherapy, which is injected into the cerebral spinal fluid. Cerebral spinal fluid actively circulates into the brain, helping to maintain the brain's shape and pressure. Delivering chemotherapy directly into the CNS is done in an attempt to prevent the cancer from spreading to the brain. However, chemotherapy is toxic to certain brain cells. Widespread reductions in brain volumes have been noted among adult survivors of leukemia, even several decades after diagnosis [9]. Survivors with lower brain volumes tend to have increased cognitive dysfunction [9].

Brain changes also occur among patients with non-CNS cancers who have not received any CNS directed therapies. One large study involved 187 chemotherapy-exposed breast cancer survivors. Compared to 374 age-matched women with no cancer history, the breast cancer survivors demonstrated significantly decreased white matter integrity throughout the brain, even 20 years after chemotherapy treatment [10].

Another study by the same research group showed reduced whole-brain **gray matter** volume, also in a large sample of breast cancer survivors [11]. Gray matter supports information processing in the brain. Studies of breast cancer survivors have also shown reduced gray matter volume in specific brain regions like the **hippocampus** [12,13], which is critical for memory, and the **prefrontal cortex**, which is important for skills like thinking and attention [14-16].

Changes in brain structure negatively affect the brain's ability to support cognitive processes. For example, studies have suggested that brain networks following breast cancer chemotherapy require involvement of more brain regions to complete certain tasks compared to healthy women [17-20]. This recruitment of additional brain resources suggests that the brain is attempting to compensate for an injury. However, the decreased efficiency associated with this compensation likely results in cognitive fatigue because the brain must work harder to do certain tasks. This compensation may cause tasks to take more time or thinking to seem slow and "foggy" because of the additional brain resources that have to be engaged. It is similar to when you take the long way or the scenic route to a destination. You will get where you are going but it takes more time and resources (e.g. gas) to get there. When the brain must use a less efficient "route" to support a certain cognitive task, it is also using more "gas" (i.e. oxygen, glucose) and may tend to get "lost" more often (i.e. make more mistakes).

Fortunately, the brain has a great deal of **neuroplasticity** and shows significant ability to recover and/or compensate from injuries. Neuroplasticity refers to the brain's ability to reorganize itself to support repair, compensation, adaptation and new learning. Neuroplasticity mechanisms are therefore critical for brain recovery. Most natural brain recovery occurs within the first one to two years following cancer and cancer treatments [21]. However, some survivors show persistent cognitive difficulties and some even show new cognitive problems that were not present earlier in their disease or treatment course [22].

It is unclear why some cancer survivors show improvement in cognitive function over time while others struggle with persistent, new or even worsening difficulties. **Neuroimaging** (brain imaging) studies involving breast cancer chemotherapy suggest that **neural compensation**, or recruitment of additional brain resources, occurs most often when task difficulty is low. As task difficulty increases, the brain may be unable to maintain this compensatory response [23], resulting in decreased brain response compared to that of similarly aged peers. Neural compensation may mask alterations in cognitive performance [23] making cognitive changes difficult to detect in some patients. These patients may obtain "normal" scores on cognitive tests despite having significant cognitive difficulties during daily living tasks.

Neural compensation also appears to be more common among patients who are pre-therapy or have been off-therapy (e.g. chemotherapy, radiation) one year or less [6,17,24,25]. Alternatively, very long-term survivors (5 or more years off-therapy) tend to show less compensatory brain activation [26,27] suggesting that this ability may decrease over time. This pattern of decreased neural compensation over time is likely due to disrupted organization of brain networks following cancer and its treatments [18,28-30]. This disruption reduces the capacity of brain networks to coordinate responses to cognitive demands.

The level of brain recovery and compensation differs significantly among patients and likely depends on several factors such as cancer type, intensity and type of cancer treatment, genetic predisposition, educational and occupational history, level of social support, age, gender, disease severity and the presence of other medical and/or psychiatric conditions. Further research is required to determine what factors or interventions might help enhance or maintain neural compensation following cancer and cancer treatments.

In summary, cognitive difficulties following cancer and/or cancer treatments are associated with measurable brain changes. Thus far, most neuroimaging research on cognitive effects following cancer has involved women with breast cancer. However, many of the mechanisms underlying the observed brain changes, such as chemotherapy and

neuroinflammation, are believed to be common across cancer types. Therefore, it is expected that individuals with other non-CNS cancers may also show brain changes. In fact, a recent study demonstrated alterations in brain metabolism during adjuvant therapy for pharyngeal cancer [31] and another study showed reduced brain activation and connectivity in patients with prostate cancer undergoing androgen deprivation therapy [32]. This means that if you are having cognitive difficulties following cancer, there is likely a biological reason. Cognitive problems are not imagined or entirely due to stress or an indication that you are "going crazy". You are also not alone. As many as 78% or more of non-CNS cancer survivors experience significant problems with cognitive skills [33,34]. This percentage is even higher for patients with brain tumor or metastasis [29]. While currently there is no standard, evidence-based treatment for these difficulties, many patients can potentially benefit from some of the interventions discussed in this book.

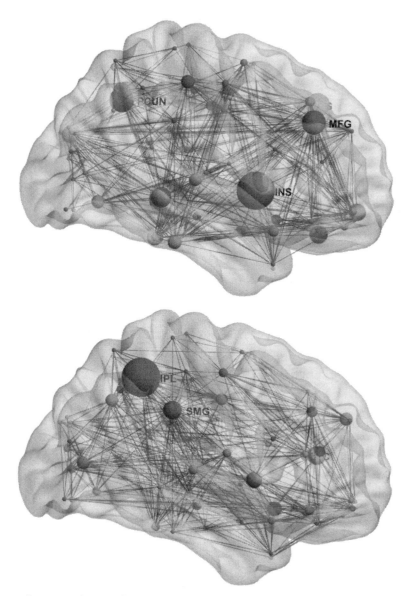

Compared to the healthy brain (top), the brain after chemotherapy (bottom) has reduced organization of brain networks (gray lines). Also, certain hub regions (large spheres) are not participating effectively in the brain network following chemotherapy. This makes the brain network less efficient (Hosseini, SMH, Koovakkattu, D & Kesler, SR. 2012. BMC Neurology, 12, 28).

Chapter 2: Mechanisms

Why do cognitive difficulties occur following cancer and its treatments? The answer to this question remains unclear but is being actively investigated. As noted previously, cognitive effects following cancer and its treatments are often referred to as chemo brain. While chemotherapy may be a major culprit in cognitive effects, there are several other factors that seem to contribute as well. Some mechanisms may be associated with certain cognitive effects but not others. Some individuals may be more vulnerable to certain mechanisms compared to others. Continued research in the area of cognition and cancer will hopefully provide more insight regarding these possibilities. Determining the mechanisms of cognitive effects following cancer is critical for developing condition-specific interventions.

Cancer Pathology

Primary brain tumors and brain metastases invade healthy brain tissue causing structural injury known as "mass effect". The tumor displaces and/or compresses healthy brain tissue. Faster growing tumors tend to cause increased cognitive dysfunction, likely because the brain cannot adapt quickly enough [29]. Tumors can also cause a rise in **intracranial pressure**. The brain is housed within the **cranium**, which is a very rigid space with a fixed volume. Any increase in the contents within the brain or cranium can result in increased intracranial pressure. A primary brain tumor or large metastasis is a space-occupying, oftentimes expanding mass that tends to increase this pressure. Increased intracranial pressure can cause edema (swelling), compression and/or displacement of brain tissue, brain herniation or restricted blood supply. These complications can result in permanent brain injury depending on their severity.

As noted previously, many patients with non-CNS cancers also show changes in brain function. These changes may occur even before adjuvant cancer treatments have begun. Other studies show that patients with higher disease severity have more cognitive difficulties [27,35]. These findings suggest that the cancer itself may be contributing to cognitive difficulties in non-CNS cancers as well. This is perhaps not surprising given that it is often difficult to concentrate or remember things when one is not feeling well. Additionally, there tends to be increased inflammation in the body as the immune system responds to the disease. Inflammation is associated with molecules known as **cytokines** and these cytokines can get into the brain and disrupt brain structure and function if chronically elevated [13,36]. Some tumors are believed to engage in a hostile take-over of immune regulation, suppressing protective immune responses to the tumor [37]. Disrupted immune system function may result in chronic inflammation that continues into remission [38]. Studies suggest that cancer survivors demonstrate elevated pro-inflammatory cytokine levels even several years post-diagnosis [13,36,38,39]. Pro-inflammatory cytokines are cytokines that promote or increase inflammation.

Surgery

Surgery is frequently used to remove a primary brain tumor or brain metastatic mass and reduce intracranial pressure. Advanced surgical technology has resulted in improved tumor removal or resection. However, this tends to involve larger volumes of brain tissue being removed, which is potentially damaging to functioning brain regions [40]. Accordingly, some patients show improvement in cognitive function following tumor resection while others show worsening of cognitive function [40,41]. The location and size of the tumor seem to significantly influence the patient's cognitive outcome following resection. Additionally, cognitive worsening following tumor resection may be only temporary [40,42].

Surgery for non-CNS cancers such as mastectomy in patients with breast cancer has also been implicated in cognitive effects [43,44]. One study examined patients with breast cancer from pre-surgery to two years after surgery. Self-rated attention declined in 54% of women and was at its lowest point one month after surgery. Attention improved to pre-surgery level over the next year despite patients undergoing adjuvant chemotherapy during that time [45]. However, it is difficult to separate the effects of anxiety from these findings especially since they relied exclusively on self-reported cognitive function.

The effects of surgery on cognitive function likely stem from general anesthesia and inflammation. General anesthesia works directly on the brain but has not historically been suspected of causing any permanent brain damage. However, emerging research suggests that brain injury may occur following general anesthesia for major surgery in some patients [46]. Cognitive effects of general anesthesia are often referred to as "postoperative cognitive dysfunction (POCD)" and are believed to be temporary, lasting less than six months in most patients [47,48]. POCD is more common in elderly patients but does occur in middle-aged patients as well [49]. Increased inflammation and pain following surgery may increase the risk for POCD [50,51].

Chemotherapy

As noted in Chapter 1, some patients receive intrathecal chemotherapy, which is delivered directly into the CNS. Chemotherapy is toxic to **neural progenitor cells**. These progenitor cells form **neurons** and other types of brain cells. Neurons are brain cells that process and transmit information. They make up the gray matter of the brain. Neurons cannot self-renew (i.e. generate new neurons) so once a neuron dies, it is gone forever. However, like other types of stem cells, neural progenitor cells can self-renew. This **self-renewal** is a critical process in the brain's ability to learn new information, reorganize itself in response to the environment and heal after injury or disease.

The brain is normally protected by the **blood-brain barrier**, which prevents many substances that are in the blood from getting into the brain. Many chemotherapeutic agents cannot actively cross the blood-brain barrier. Therefore, the notion of chemo brain in patients who receive **systemic chemotherapy** has been somewhat controversial in the past. Systemic chemotherapy is typically delivered intravenously (i.e. IV) or orally (e.g. pills) - not directly into the CNS. However, disease states such as cancer may make the blood-brain barrier more permeable to chemotherapy and other toxins [1,52,53].

There is increasing evidence that at least some systemic chemotherapy is entering the brain. These studies indicate that neural progenitor cells lose their capacity for self-renewal, even after an initial dose of systemic chemotherapy [54]. Repeated doses cause persistent suppression of self-renewal [54-56]. Therefore, even small amounts of chemotherapy getting into the brain may be sufficient to cause significant damage [56-61]. Damage to brain progenitor cells disrupts neuroplasticity mechanisms [56], which are vital for learning, memory and adaptation of the brain's responses to the changing environment.

Chemotherapy may cause indirect brain injury by elevating inflammation. Several common chemotherapies have been shown to elevate pro-inflammatory cytokine levels [62-65]. Cytokines actively cross the blood-brain barrier [66] and also indirectly lead to impairment of blood-brain barrier integrity [67-69]. Elevated cytokine levels can be toxic to brain cells. They can stimulate local inflammation and are associated with damage from **oxidative stress**, which disrupts communication between cells [70-75]. Oxidative stress occurs when the products of oxygen metabolism, or breakdown, become out of balance, resulting in a toxic cellular environment.

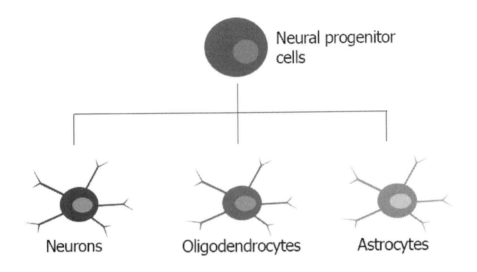

Neurons, oligodendrocytes and astrocytes are types of brain cells. These brain cells all come from neural progenitor cells. Neurons are responsible for information processing and make up the gray matter of the brain. Oligodendrocytes help form myelin, which is important for white matter development. Astrocytes support neurons as well as the cells in the blood-brain barrier. Normally, neural progenitor cells can self-renew but chemotherapy suppresses this ability.

Chemotherapy may also result in **DNA** damage that negatively affects brain structure and function [53]. DNA contains our genetic blueprint. Our genes provide information for the formation of proteins that play certain critical roles in various systems throughout the body, including the brain. When DNA is affected, these proteins may become altered and less effective. Certain chemotherapies target cancer cells by breaking DNA and unfortunately this DNA damage can extend to healthy cells as well [53]. Also, as noted above, chemotherapy can induce oxidative stress, which is harmful to DNA [76]. Oxidative stress is the most common cause of DNA damage in neurons [53]. Oxidative DNA damage has been shown to be higher in patients following chemotherapy and is associated with brain alterations in these patients [77].

As we get older, various changes occur within the brain including loss of gray matter, reduction of white matter pathway integrity, increased protein deposits, altered neurochemical levels and variations in gene expression, among others. These brain changes are often associated with normal declines in cognitive functions including decreased memory, processing speed, executive function and attention.

There is some evidence that chemotherapy may accelerate this brain aging process. Cancer survivors who are older tend to have poorer cognitive outcome following chemotherapy [27,78]. Also, many of the brain changes associated with chemotherapy treatment overlap with those observed in brain aging. Specifically, one study suggested that reductions in gray matter volume following chemotherapy treatment correspond to approximately four years of aging on the brain [11].

Several studies have shown abnormalities in default mode network brain regions following chemotherapy [13-15,18,19,79,80]. The default mode network is a brain network that supports important processes such as incidental learning, autobiographical memory retrieval, foresight, monitoring and other internally focused thought processes [81]. Change in default mode network connectivity is a significant marker of healthy as well as **pathological** age-related cognitive decline

[82]. One study demonstrated that abnormality of default mode network connectivity may be highly specific to chemotherapy treatment while alternate brain networks might be more sensitive to other cancer treatments [83].

Chemotherapy-treated breast cancer survivors also demonstrate altered levels of neurochemicals in the brain. Specifically, they may show significantly increased levels of **myo-inositol** and **choline** as well as decreased **N-acetylaspartate**/myo-inositol and N-acetylaspartate/choline ratios in the brain compared to healthy women [84]. This same neurochemical profile is associated with aging [85] and is highly predictive of pathological age-related cognitive decline [86]. Another study showed that approximately 30% of patients treated with chemotherapy showed a new onset of previously non-existent cognitive decline [22]. Therefore, cognitive function may actually worsen over time in some patients.

If chemotherapy does accelerate brain aging, there is some concern that it may increase the risk for **dementia** (e.g. **Alzheimer's disease**). One study of 18,360 women with breast cancer showed that those treated with chemotherapy were 1.2 times more likely to have dementia during long-term follow-up [87]. However, a subsequent study of 62,565 women failed to replicate this finding [88] and therefore the association between dementia and chemotherapy remains controversial. It is perhaps more likely that chemotherapy-treated patients fall somewhere between normal and pathological aging in terms of cognitive decline. Alternatively, chemotherapy may increase the risk for dementia only in patients who already have other risk factors such as specific genetic markers [78]. In fact, one study showed that while brain resilience to simulated aging was reduced in chemotherapy treated breast cancer survivors, it was not accelerated compared to healthy controls [89]. Early intervention including regular cognitive and physical activity, surveillance of cognitive function over time and ongoing stress management is critical for helping to prevent further cognitive decline (see Chapters 4-9).

Radiation

Cranial radiation is a significant risk factor for long-term cognitive impairments [90]. **Radiation necrosis** is a side effect of cranial and neck radiotherapy that occurs in some patients. It is associated with lesions, swelling and degradation of brain tissue. Radiation necrosis is believed to result from increased cytokine levels (inflammation), increased capillary leakage, edema (swelling), **myelin** damage and release of vascular endothelial growth factor (VEGF) [91-93]. VEGF is a protein associated with the creation of new blood vessels. In disease states, the overexpression or elevation of VEGF often results in abnormal blood vessels that interfere with normal physiologic functions. Radiation to the head or neck can also accelerate atherosclerosis (hardening of artery walls) and increase the risk of future stroke [31].

Cranial radiation also disrupts **neurogenesis** (creation of new neurons) in the hippocampus. Research indicates that radiation therapy results in increased cell death, decreased **cell proliferation** (growth) and decreased **cell differentiation** (development into neurons) in the hippocampus [94]. One study demonstrated that new neuron production was decreased by 97% in the hippocampus just two months following a single cranial radiation dose [93]. Additional radiation doses result in increasing neural progenitor cell damage [93]. Cranial radiation may suppress oligodendrocyte proliferation leading to white matter necrosis [95]. Cranial radiation may also accelerate brain aging and increase risk for dementia [96].

Local radiation does not appear to affect the brain as significantly or directly as cranial radiation. However, some cognitive effects have been observed in patients who have undergone local radiotherapy alone (without chemotherapy) [4,97,98]. The mechanisms underlying cognitive effects associated with local radiotherapy remain unclear. However, local radiotherapy has been shown to have several consequences for non-irradiated cells that could impact brain function. Irradiated cells may transmit danger signals to non-irradiated cells that result in DNA damage and cell death to the non-irradiated cells [99]. Local radiotherapy can also increase inflammation [99].

Hormonal Therapies

Hormonal blockade therapies target estrogen and testosterone production resulting in reduced levels of these hormones. Estrogen and testosterone interact with brain systems to support brain function. Decreased levels of these hormones may be associated with cognitive decline.

Research regarding the effects of tamoxifen, an estrogen blockade medication, remains inconclusive. Some studies have suggested that tamoxifen is associated with cognitive difficulties, particularly in verbal memory [100-105]. However, other studies have shown no association between tamoxifen and cognitive function [13,15,22,84,106]. One study demonstrated that women taking tamoxifen had lower hippocampal volumes compared to controls [107]. On the other hand, tamoxifen has been associated with reduced myo-inositol levels suggesting that tamoxifen may be beneficial and could reduce effects of brain aging [108].

Patients with prostate cancer who undergo androgen deprivation therapy (ADT) may show difficulties with spatial reasoning and working memory [109]. ADT reduces testosterone. During a spatial task, patients with prostate cancer treated with ADT showed reduced activation of right parietal-occipital regions compared to controls [110]. A larger study of men with prostate cancer demonstrated an association between ADT and lower prefrontal cortex function and connectivity at six months post-ADT [32].

Chemotherapy can induce early menopause in women resulting in reduced estrogen levels. Therefore, even if hormonal blockade medication is not used, changes in hormone levels may also contribute to cognitive difficulties in patients who receive chemotherapy. Some studies suggest that patients treated with both chemotherapy and tamoxifen showed the greatest cognitive difficulties [101,111].

Genetic Vulnerability

Certain genetic factors may be associated with increased or decreased vulnerability to cognitive effects following cancer. These are not genetic abnormalities but normal genetic variations that are associated with normal differences in gene expression. Typically these variations do not have noticeable effects on an individual until an injury or illness occurs. Not everyone shows cognitive decline following cancer or its treatments and genetic variations may help identify subgroups of patients who are at higher risk for cognitive effects.

APOE is a gene that regulates the build-up of a protein called amyloid beta. Increased accumulation of amyloid beta in the brain is associated with Alzheimer's disease and is therefore believed to negatively impact brain and cognitive function. The APOE gene has six different genotype combinations. Each genotype is associated with different levels of amyloid beta accumulation with the E4 variant being associated with the most accumulation [112,113]. The E4 variant occurs in approximately 15% of the population and is a significant risk factor for Alzheimer's disease [114]. Patients with the E4 genotype show worse outcome following traumatic brain injury compared to patients with other APOE genotypes [115]. The risk associated with APOE4 appears to be dose-dependent - individuals can have zero, one or two E4 **alleles** on the APOE gene and increasing number of E4 alleles is associated with increasing risk.

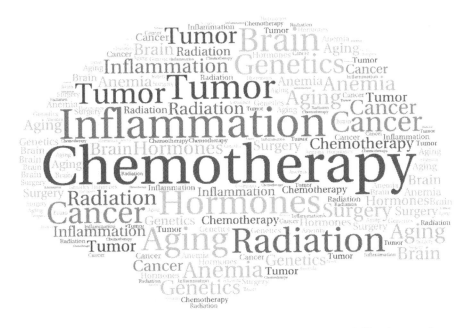

There are several possible reasons for cognitive difficulties after cancer. Research in this area is still very new and some potential mechanisms such as chemotherapy have received more research attention than others such as surgery or anemia. These candidate mechanisms likely interact with each other and/or amplify one another. There could also be other factors that contribute to cognitive difficulties that are currently unknown.

Because chemotherapy is believed to result in brain injury and brain aging, the APOE4 genotype may increase the risk for chemotherapy-related cognitive difficulties as well. One study examined cognitive function in 80 chemotherapy-treated survivors of breast cancer or lymphoma. Survivors with the presence of an E4 allele showed reduced performance on measures of visual memory, spatial ability and processing speed compared to those without any E4 alleles [116]. These results suggest that APOE4 may be a risk factor for certain cognitive difficulties but not others. Accordingly, another study did not find any association between APOE4 and executive function [16].

Variation in the COMT gene has also been linked with poorer cognitive outcome, particularly on measures of word finding, attention and motor speed, following chemotherapy treatment [117]. COMT is associated with dopamine levels in the prefrontal cortex. Dopamine is a **neurotransmitter** that is significantly involved in cognitive function. The Val variation of COMT is associated with reduced dopamine availability and even healthy carriers of this allele show decreased performance on measures of attention and executive function compared to individuals with the Met genotype [118].

Other genotype variations have been proposed as possible risk factors for cancer and/or treatment-related cognitive deficits [78]. These include BDNF, which is important for neuroplasticity and MDR1, which plays a role in blood-brain barrier function. Genes that influence inflammation such as IL-6 may also be involved. However, research studies of these genes and their relationship to cognitive effects following cancer have not yet been conducted.

Anemia

Anemia is associated with reduced cognitive function in patients with cancer [119-121] and also in healthy adults [122]. Anemia refers to a lack of healthy red blood cells. Red blood cells carry oxygen and therefore, anemia tends to result in reduced oxygen delivery to body tissues. The brain is the largest consumer of oxygen in the body, requiring approximately 20% of the total oxygen supply. Therefore, the brain is highly sensitive to fluctuations in oxygen levels and reduced oxygen levels can disrupt brain function. Additionally anemia tends to cause significant fatigue. It is estimated that 30-90% of patients with cancer are affected by anemia depending on the cancer diagnosis and the definition of anemia [119].

One study examined 88 patients with acute myelogenous leukemia or myelodysplastic syndrome. Study findings indicated decreased cognitive functioning in patients with hemoglobin levels of 10 g/dL or below. Word finding, attention, and fine motor function were the most affected cognitive skills [121]. Anemia also increases the risk for delirium in patients undergoing bone marrow transplant [123]. Delirium refers to a state of severe confusion and disorientation indicating that the brain has been negatively affected.

Anemia can result from destruction of red blood cells, blood loss and/or impaired red blood cell production [119]. Tumors and chemotherapy can destroy red blood cells and disrupt red blood cell production. Hormones, including testosterone and estrogen, play important roles in the production of red blood cells and therefore hormonal blockade treatments are also associated with anemia [124-126].

Other Medications

Patients with cancer often receive a number of additional medications during their treatment. Examples include corticosteroids, antiemetics, antivirals, antibiotics, appetite stimulants, sedatives and pain medications. Some of these drugs work by affecting the brain. However, it is largely unknown if these medications contribute to cognitive difficulties. They could have independent effects and/or could interact with other cancer treatments. Further research in this area is needed.

In summary, there are several possible explanations for cognitive difficulties following cancer and cancer treatments. These include mass effect, suppression of neural progenitor cells, acceleration of brain aging, inflammation, altered hormone levels, blood vessel damage, DNA damage, anemia and genetic predisposition. There are some mechanisms like inflammation, anemia and genetic predisposition that are likely common across cancer diagnoses while other mechanisms such as cranial radiation and mass effect are specific to certain cancers. Some mechanisms seem to affect certain brain regions and therefore certain cognitive skills more so than others. Much of the research that has been conducted to date has focused on a particular mechanism at the exclusion of others. However, it is possible and perhaps even likely that cognitive difficulties following cancer result from an interaction between and/or a collective effect of multiple mechanisms. There could also be other important mechanisms that are currently unknown.

Chapter 3: Cognitive Functions

The most frequently observed cognitive difficulties following cancer and its treatments include declines in executive functioning, memory, attention and processing speed [22,33]. However, difficulties in other cognitive areas are also possible. There is significant variation among patients in terms of the types of difficulties that occur and how much these difficulties interfere with daily living tasks.

Executive Function

Executive function refers to a set of cognitive skills that is critical for adaptation and goal-oriented behaviors. There are core executive functions including working memory, response inhibition and cognitive flexibility. **Working memory** refers to the short-term storage and manipulation of information. Individuals with working memory difficulties struggle with multi-tasking and often forget or lose track of what they were doing or thinking. They may have trouble with reading since reading requires storage of context and passage meaning in short-term memory as the individual continues to read. Conversations may be difficult to track and word finding problems may occur. Working memory is a critical element of general intelligence and a key component in a wide range of other cognitive skills.

Response inhibition is the suppression of actions that interfere with goal-directed behaviors. Individuals with deficits in response inhibition may struggle with impulsivity, delaying responses, remaining on task, resisting distraction and/or switching from one task or train of thought to another. **Cognitive flexibility** is the ability to generate multiple alternative solutions to problems and switch fluidly between thoughts or actions. Individuals with impairment in cognitive flexibility tend to get stuck when trying to solve problems. They may have trouble recognizing that there is more than one answer or approach to a certain task and that their response may not be the best one. They may have difficulty realizing when they have made mistakes as a result. Deficits in cognitive flexibility can also manifest as difficulty adapting to changes or "letting go" of things.

Other executive skills including planning, initiation, task monitoring, organization, self-regulation and self-control tend to stem from these core executive functions. Like the executive of a company, executive functions are required for management and coordination of behaviors. Executive function difficulties can affect other skills including memory and social functioning. Executive function problems are often the most debilitating for patients since they tend to disrupt social, home, occupational and educational functioning. Patients with executive function difficulties tend to make more mistakes in managing their cancer medications [127] and may struggle with health behaviors such as physical activity and diet [128-130].

Several brain regions, primarily the prefrontal cortex, support executive function. Neuroimaging studies have demonstrated abnormalities in the prefrontal cortex following cancer and its treatments. These changes are noted early on (i.e. before adjuvant chemotherapy) as well as in long-term survivors (10 years off therapy or more) [5,25-27]. The prefrontal cortex is a region of high neuroplasticity and has unique neurochemical and metabolic properties that might make it more vulnerable to chemotherapy [131,132]. The prefrontal cortex also contains numerous estrogen and androgen receptors, which might make it particularly vulnerable to hormonal blockade treatments. Patients with executive function difficulties may show a wide range of difficulties. Here a list of some common symptoms that may indicate executive function difficulties:

Speaking or acting without thinking

Trouble concentrating

Difficulty persisting with a task or following through

Difficulty figuring out how to begin a task or what approach to take

Difficulty doing more than one thing at a time (multi-tasking)

Being easily overwhelmed

Difficulties with decision-making

Losing track of what one is doing

Personal spaces, belongings and/or materials are disorganized

Frequently over-reacting and/or showing poor tolerance for frustration

Often being unprepared or lost

Difficulty thinking of alternative solutions to a problem

Tending to repeat the same response even when it is incorrect

Not realizing when a mistake has been made

Memory

The ability to recall information is critical for our daily functioning and quality of life. Memory involves several steps, including encoding, storage and retrieval. During encoding, information is received, processed and integrated. Encoding requires active attention to the information and filtering out of distracting or irrelevant information. Memory storage includes a sensory store that is very brief, less than a second, and involves simply having a perception of the information. Short-term memory storage lasts for approximately 20-30 seconds and can hold an average of seven pieces of information. Long-term memory represents a permanent record and can be enhanced through rehearsal, organizational strategies or strong emotion. Retrieval refers to recollection of stored information.

Forgetting can occur due to problems in any of these stages – encoding, storage and/or retrieval. A person may be distracted during the encoding process or may have difficulty accurately perceiving or organizing the information. Retrieval failures can occur when the memory is adequately stored but cannot be recalled due to changes in context or cues that the memory depends on. Forgetting can also occur due to interference from other information. Proactive interference occurs when previously learned information interferes with the learning of new information. Retroactive interference occurs when new information interferes with the recollection of previously learned information. Some patients forget certain information due to psychological factors such as repression of painful memories. Some memories might decay over time for reasons that remain unclear. There are several different types of memory:

Declarative/explicit memory: information learned through conscious attention

Procedural memory: actions, skills or operations

Implicit memory: information learned incidentally or without conscious attention

Autobiographical memory: life experiences

Cancer and cancer treatments tend to most commonly affect declarative memory although some patients experience difficulties in other types of memory as well.

Memory relies on several brain regions including the prefrontal cortex and the hippocampus. The hippocampus is a small structure located within the temporal lobe of the brain. Several studies have demonstrated reduced hippocampal volumes following cancer and chemotherapy. Lower hippocampal volumes are associated with lower scores on memory tests [12,13,107].

The hippocampus is unique in that it is one of the only sources of neural stem cells throughout the lifespan. This also makes it particularly vulnerable to chemotherapeutic agents because these medications show a stronger preference for progenitor cells than for cancer cells [56].

The hippocampus also has abundant cytokine receptors and may therefore be especially vulnerable to inflammation. In fact, reduced hippocampal volume has been associated with elevated pro-inflammatory cytokine levels following chemotherapy [13]. Like the prefrontal cortex, the hippocampus also contains numerous estrogen and androgen receptors. Lower hippocampal volumes have been noted in patients who have received tamoxifen, a hormonal blockade medication [107].

Attention

Focusing or concentrating on specific tasks or information can be difficult following cancer and its treatments. Being easily distracted, forgetful and losing track of what one is doing are often signs of attention difficulties. Poor organizational skills, frequent errors and difficulty listening are also associated with attention problems. There are different types of attention. Sustained attention or vigilance refers to the ability to focus on something for an extended period of time. Selective attention is the ability to focus on relevant information while ignoring irrelevant information. Divided or dual attention is the ability to focus on more than one thing at time.

The prefrontal cortex participates in some of the brain networks involved in attention. The parietal cortex is another region of the brain that supports attention processes. Neuroimaging studies have demonstrated reduction of white

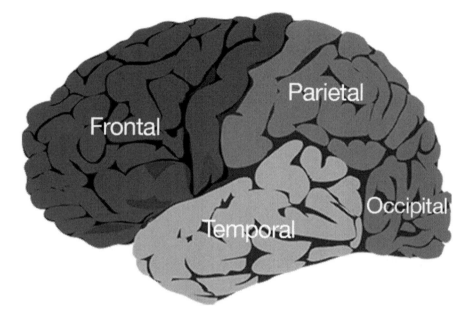

The brain is divided into several regions called lobes. The frontal lobe is important for preparing complex behaviors including executive functions, attention, memory, motor responses and emotional responses. The parietal lobe is responsible for spatial processing, sensory-perception, working memory and attention. The temporal lobe supports language, memory and visual perception. The hippocampus, a structure critical for memory, is located within the temporal lobe. The occipital lobe contains the primary visual cortex, which supports vision.

matter pathway integrity in the parietal regions in cancer survivors [79,80,133,134]. Lower parietal white matter integrity is associated with lower scores on measures of attention in chemotherapy-treated patients [134]. White matter pathways consist of myelinated fibers that link various areas of the brain together. These pathways are critical for communication between and coordination of different specialized brain regions.

White matter pathways provide the structure or backbone for functional brain networks. These various networks support cognitive processes such as learning and memory, executive function, language and visual-spatial processing, among others. As noted in Chapter 2, chemotherapy can be toxic to neural progenitor cells, including those that form **oligodendrocytes**. Oligodendrocytes are important for white matter myelination. Myelin provides a type of insulation around the part of a neuron called the axon. Myelin allows a neuron to communicate more rapidly with other neurons.

Processing Speed

Processing speed, or reaction time, refers to how quickly the brain can process information. Many cancer survivors describe their thinking as being slow or foggy. Mental processes seem inefficient and tasks take longer to accomplish than before. These symptoms are consistent with reduced cognitive processing speed. Processing speed tends to worsen when tasks are more difficult or complex or when distractions are present. Any tasks that must be completed under time pressure will be difficult. Slowing in processing speed can result in difficulties with other cognitive functions such as memory or executive control. Attention problems can worsen processing speed.

Processing speed relies largely on the prefrontal cortex as well as connectivity between various brain regions. This connectivity depends upon the integrity of white matter pathways. As noted above, these pathways consist of myelinated fibers and myelin significantly increases communication speed between neurons. Thus, damage to white matter integrity would slow down this communication among brain regions. Lower scores on tests of processing speed have been associated with the reduction of white matter integrity in cancer survivors [79,135].

In summary, cognitive skills such as memory, executive function, attention and processing speed are controlled by the brain. Specific cognitive skills arise from the coordination of certain specialized brain regions within functional brain networks. These functional networks rely on white matter pathways. Cognitive difficulties can result from alteration or injury to one or more of these specialized regions and/or to the pathways that connect these regions. Thus far, it seems that prefrontal cortex, hippocampus and white matter pathways are particularly vulnerable to cancer and cancer treatments.

Chapter 4: Clinical Care

If you are experiencing difficulties with cognitive abilities such as problems with memory, thinking, attention, etc., that are interfering with your daily functioning, you should consider consulting with your doctor for appropriate clinical care referrals. This chapter provides information regarding clinical evaluation and treatment for cognitive difficulties following cancer. These procedures require the involvement of a health or mental health clinician. Chapters 5 through 9 provide information regarding potential interventions that you can do independently.

Evaluation

A **neuropsychological evaluation** is the standard of care for any individual who has experienced a potential change in brain function. A licensed psychologist who has specialty training and experience in **neuropsychology** - the study of brain-behavior relationships, conducts these evaluations. The evaluation typically consists of an interview and several hours of testing. During the interview, the neuropsychologist will ask you questions about your background including your academic and occupational achievements and your medical history. It is helpful to come prepared with copies of any medical records you might have. A list of medications that you are currently taking is also useful. The neuropsychologist will also ask you about your symptoms, how long you have been experiencing them and how they affect your daily functioning. The neuropsychologist might ask to talk with your significant other or additional people who can provide insight regarding your background and cognitive difficulties.

During the testing portion of the evaluation, the neuropsychologist and/or a trained technician will administer multiple tests to you. These tests will measure various brain functions including intelligence, memory, problem solving, processing speed, sensory-perception, motor skills, language, academic skills and attention. Tests might also include measures of psychiatric symptoms including **depression** and **anxiety**. Testing might include measures administered via computer. The testing process will require several hours but can be broken up over more than one session if necessary.

The goal of the evaluation is to obtain your very best cognitive performance. This may seem counterintuitive since your main concern is what to do about your cognitive *difficulties*. However, some cognitive failures tend to occur during settings where there are many distractions or when you are stressed or tired. These factors can be altered so it is more important to know what cognitive difficulties you have during optimal conditions. These difficulties will typically be the most debilitating and require the greatest emphasis in your treatment planning.

Therefore, try to avoid scheduling your neuropsychological testing during times that you know you will be more tired. If you become fatigued easily, you should consult with the neuropsychologist about completing the tests at times of the day when you are more alert and also consider breaking up the testing session over several days. Reschedule your testing appointment if you become ill, even with a common cold. Refrain from taking any sedative type medications on the day of the evaluation as these can affect your cognitive performance. If you are experiencing significant physical pain, take necessary steps to manage this appropriately so that it does not interfere with your testing. Be sure to tell the neuropsychologist or technician if you need a break during testing.

After your testing is complete, the neuropsychologist will review all the information and formulate an evaluation report. The report could take several weeks depending on how many patients the neuropsychologist has. After the report is completed, the neuropsychologist will meet with you and discuss the results. The report should include a treatment plan for addressing your difficulties. The neuropsychologist will explain this treatment plan to you and provide suggestions for obtaining the services that you need. You should be prepared to take notes and ask questions to make sure that you understand what the neuropsychologist tells you. You may want to bring a significant other, friend or family member with you to help. Sometimes a spouse or family member can help you think of questions to ask that you might not think of yourself.

Because cognitive difficulties following cancer can worsen over time in some patients, it is beneficial to have a neuropsychological evaluation regularly. Additionally, as described in Chapter 1, neural compensation can make cognitive changes difficult to detect in some patients. Repeated assessment is often necessary to determine a patient's relative decline in cognitive function. Generally, the recommendation is for re-evaluation every one to two years although your neuropsychologist will specify this for you. It is recommended that you track your cognitive function over time to ensure that any changes are detected early so that any necessary interventions can be put into place.

Most major health insurance benefits provide coverage for neuropsychological evaluations, although some require preauthorization. You can ask your insurance company if they cover neuropsychological evaluation (CPT codes 96118 and 96119). The evaluation is typically insured under mental health benefits but could alternatively involve your medical benefit since the cognitive difficulties are considered related to your medical diagnosis, depending on your insurance. Sometimes you must do a diagnostic evaluation before your insurance will agree to cover the neuropsychological evaluation. The diagnostic evaluation involves an interview with the neuropsychologist during which your symptoms are discussed. The neuropsychologist must then complete paperwork to justify continuing with the evaluation and doing testing. This paperwork is submitted to your insurance company who then decides whether or not to proceed.

Treatment

There currently is no specific treatment or cure for cancer-related cognitive difficulties. Such treatments are still being investigated and developed. As research regarding the mechanisms of cancer-related cognitive difficulties continues to advance, more progress in the area of interventions will be made. This section discusses some of the past and present research regarding possible treatments for cancer-related cognitive effects. However, none of these interventions are condition-specific meaning that none of them were designed to exclusively treat cancer-related cognitive effects. Rather, they are interventions that could be used to treat cognitive difficulties associated with a wide variety of conditions.

Therefore, these interventions may only address certain symptoms and/or may only be moderately effective. This lack of specificity is due in part to the tremendous complexity involved in treating cognitive difficulties. Cognition is based in the brain and the brain is the most complex system in the known universe. The brain has over 100 billion neurons and 100 trillion connections! Understanding how the brain works is an ongoing challenge but one of very high priority (e.g. http://www.whitehouse.gov/infographics/brain-initiative).

Medications that target regions of the brain that are injured following cancer and cancer treatments may help alleviate certain cognitive symptoms. There is some evidence that modafinil may help improve memory, attention and fatigue in cancer survivors with various diagnoses, including brain tumor [136,137]. Modafinil is a stimulant medication that is believed to affect the neurochemistry of the prefrontal cortex

[138,139]. In one study, 82 women with breast cancer received 200 milligrams of modafinil once a day for four weeks. Patients who showed a positive response were then randomly assigned to an additional four weeks of modafinil or a **placebo**. Modafinil was associated with improvements in memory and attention [136].

In another study, 28 cancer patients with various cancer diagnoses were randomly assigned to receive a single 200 milligram dose of modafinil or a placebo. Patients who received modafinil demonstrated significantly improved motor speed, attention, mood and fatigue [137]. Another stimulant medication, methylphenidate, has also been associated with improved cognitive function in cancer patients, especially when combined with physical exercise [140].

Early evidence suggests that bevacizumab may be effective for reducing radiation necrosis [91]. As described in Chapter 2, radiation may be associated with the release of VEGF in the brain, which can impair the blood-brain barrier and cause swelling [91]. Bevacizumab inhibits VEGF.

Several studies have examined the effects of estrogen supplement (estradiol) on cognitive function following prostate cancer and indicate promising preliminary results [141]. Estrogen supplement aims to help normalize hormone levels that have been depleted by hormonal suppression therapies. One study examined the effects of plant estrogen, such as that found in soybeans, on cognitive function in patients with prostate cancer. Unfortunately, there were no significant results but this may have been due to the small number of patients in the study [142].

Medications like modafinil, methylphenidate, bevacizumab or estradiol must be prescribed by a physician and potential side effects should be carefully discussed and considered. For example, stimulant medications may be associated with insomnia. Cancer survivors are at increased risk for insomnia and therefore you should be sure to inform your doctor if you have insomnia or other sleeping difficulties when considering stimulant medications. Additionally, estrogen supplements have been associated with increased risk of heart attack, stroke and dementia in women [141].

Cognitive rehabilitation is a behavioral method that is used to help improve cognitive difficulties. Cognitive rehabilitation has historically been used mostly in patients with traumatic brain injury or stroke. However, its effectiveness in other syndromes has been demonstrated during the past few decades. This intervention typically involves meeting with a trained clinician for several sessions during which cognitive strategies and skills are taught. The number and duration of these sessions varies widely but you can expect to meet with the therapist at least once per week for 30-60 minutes. The total number of sessions also varies and depends largely on your individual treatment plan.

Some cognitive rehabilitation approaches involve family members, home visits by the therapist and/or workplace-specific interventions. The treatment plan typically relies very heavily on homework assignments including regular and intensive practice of cognitive and stress management skills. Cognitive rehabilitation is conducted by neuropsychologists, occupational therapists and speech/language pathologists. Neuropsychologists can additionally address any significant psychiatric difficulties that are present, such as depression and anxiety. Occupational therapists can focus on work- or home-specific cognitive skills and strategies.

Ferguson and colleagues demonstrated that a brief cognitive rehabilitation program focused on management of cognitive difficulties could be effective for improving memory in cancer survivors [143,144]. The most recent study involved 40 female breast cancer survivors who were at least 18 months off-therapy. Participants were randomly assigned to the treatment group or a waitlist group. The intervention required four biweekly individual office visits that were 30–50 minutes in duration. These sessions were conducted by a clinical psychologist. Participants were provided with a workbook that included homework assignments for cognitive strategies, self-monitoring and stress management. Results indicated improved well-being, quality of life and verbal memory in the treatment group compared to the waitlist group.

One study randomly assigned 140 patients with glioma who had been medically stable for at least six months to a cognitive rehabilitation group or a waitlist group. The rehabilitation program consisted of six weekly, two hour sessions of computer-based attention skills practice and compensatory skills training focusing on attention, memory, and executive functioning. Sessions were conducted by neuropsychologists. Results indicated that, compared to the waitlist group, the rehab group demonstrated significant improvement in attention, verbal memory and fatigue [145].

Another study examined the effectiveness of cognitive rehabilitation in 58 patients with primary brain tumor. Patients were randomly assigned to a rehabilitation group or a control group. The rehabilitation program consisted of 16, one-hour sessions involving therapist-guided cognitive skill and strategy training. The program lasted for four weeks. Compared to the control group, patients enrolled in the rehabilitation group demonstrated significant improvement in cognitive function, especially in visual attention and verbal memory [146].

Unfortunately, cognitive rehabilitation is not always widely available or covered by health insurance. You can ask your insurance provider if cognitive rehabilitation therapy is among your benefits (CPT code 97532). Occupational therapy involves separate CPT codes (97535 - 97537). A neuropsychological evaluation will typically include recommendations for cognitive rehabilitation if it is appropriate for you.

Prognosis

Predicting which patients are at highest risk for persistent and/or worsening cognitive decline would be invaluable for treatment decision-making as well as implementing early intervention. Unfortunately, reliable prognostic indicators are not currently available. It seems that older age, higher disease stage, certain genetic variations and lower education level are associated with poorer cognitive outcome. However, there currently are no established cut-off points for these parameters. For example, at what specific age or age range do patients become significantly vulnerable for persistent cognitive difficulties? Continued research regarding cognition and cancer will hopefully provide more specific predictors.

One very promising method for predicting cognitive outcome following cancer involves the combination of neuroimaging with artificial intelligence. Neuroimaging is a method of viewing and measuring various aspects of the brain including volume, white matter integrity, functional activity and metabolism, among others. Magnetic resonance imaging (MRI) and positron emission tomography (PET) scans are examples of neuroimaging techniques.

Machine learning is a type of artificial intelligence. It is a computer program that can learn by example. By providing a machine learning program with examples of neuroimaging data from various groups, it can find a pattern of brain structure and/or function that reliably and accurately distinguishes between different disease states or conditions. This allows clinical scientists to predict outcomes for individual patients, such as disease progression, based on the patient's particular brain profile. The use of machine learning and neuroimaging has been shown to be more accurate in predicting cognitive outcome than behavioral factors [147].

One study used machine learning to determine a pattern of brain network connectivity that could accurately distinguish between chemotherapy and non-chemotherapy treated breast cancer survivors. The study used MRI to measure brain network connectivity. The chemotherapy group demonstrated significant cognitive difficulties whereas the non-chemotherapy group did not. The results demonstrated that chemotherapy treated breast cancer survivors could be distinguished from non-chemotherapy treated survivors with 91% accuracy [83]. Additionally, the machine learning pattern was significantly associated with memory function. With further refinement, this method could be applied to a pre-treatment MRI scan to predict cognitive outcome at long-term follow up. Pre-treatment MRI scans are not currently part of the standard of care for most cancers other than brain tumor. However, with continued research support and development, this prognostic tool could be implemented in the near future.

In summary, if you are experiencing significant cognitive difficulties that interfere with your ability to perform daily living tasks, it is recommended that you undergo a neuropsychological evaluation. This evaluation will provide an assessment of your cognitive strengths and weaknesses and also prescribe a treatment plan. Treatments may include medication, cognitive rehabilitation or other recommendations for helping to address cognitive limitations. Research methods including machine learning are being developed to help determine the prognosis of individual patients in terms of cognitive outcome.

Chapter 5: Cognitive Exercise

There are many strategies that you can try on your own that can potentially improve cognitive function, in addition to any recommendations that your neuropsychologist might make. One important approach is cognitive exercise. The brain works very much like a muscle. It becomes stronger and more efficient with regular exercise.

Cognitive Training

Cognitive training involves a structured program of brain exercises that are typically presented in a game-like format. These exercises are designed to practice cognitive skills and engage brain regions that support these cognitive skills. In physical exercise, muscles and the cardiovascular system will eventually adapt to the exercise and therefore, the intensity of the workout. The same is true for the brain. The brain will quickly adapt or habituate and therefore cognitive training exercises become more difficult as you progress.

It can be very stressful to experience cognitive failures during daily activities. Cognitive exercises allow you to practice cognitive tasks in a safe, low stress environment, at your own pace. Multiple research studies have shown that cognitive training results in improved brain structure and function in non-cancer populations [148-155]. One very large study involving 620 healthyadults age 50 and older demonstrated significant improvements in cognitive function following only 10 hours of cognitive training [156]. This study used a commercially available visual speed of processing program created by Posit Science (http://www.positscience.com/). Participants who completed the at-home training were estimated to have gained 2.3 to 5.9 years of protection against age-related cognitive decline [156]. Given that chemotherapy may accelerate brain aging (see Chapter 2), this potential protection may be very important for cancer survivors.

Accordingly, cognitive training has recently been investigated in cancer survivors [157,158]. During one study, 41 female breast cancer survivors were randomly assigned to either an active training group or a waitlist group. Both groups completed several neuropsychological tests at the beginning of the study. The 21 women assigned to the training group then completed 12 weeks of cognitive training. The online training program was done entirely at home and required approximately 20-30 minutes, four days per week. Both groups were then re-tested. Results indicated that, compared to the waitlist group, the active group showed improvements in executive function, word finding, memory and processing speed. The active group also rated themselves as having reduced executive function problems as well as reduced depression [158]. This study used Lumosity (http://www.lumosity.com) for the cognitive training program. The specific training schedule involved five exercises per day, four days per week. The order of the exercises is listed below:

Sessions 1-20: Brain Shift, By the Rules, Disillusion (odd sessions) or Penguin Pursuit (even sessions), Route to Sprout, Word Bubbles (odd sessions) or Color Match (even sessions)

Sessions 21-24: Brain Shift Overdrive, By the Rules, Disillusion (odd sessions) or Penguin Pursuit (even sessions), Route to Sprout, Word Bubbles (odd sessions) or Color Match (even sessions)

Sessions 25-44: Memory Matrix, Memory Match, Money Comb, Familiar Faces, Top Chimp

Sessions 45-48: Memory Matrix, Memory Match Overdrive, Money Comb, Familiar Faces, Top Chimp

Another study demonstrated that Posit Science's InSight program was effective for improving processing speed in cancer survivors [157]. In this study, 82 breast cancer survivors were randomly assigned to one of three groups: memory training, InSight processing speed training or a waitlist. All three interventions involved ten, 60 minute, in-person training sessions completed in small groups of three to five participants. The study interventions were conducted over six to eight weeks and administered by trained and certified

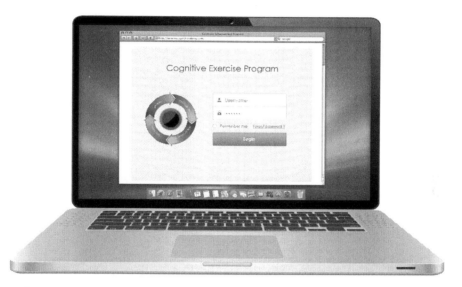

Playing computerized cognitive exercises or "brain games" may help improve cognitive function. These games allow you to practice different cognitive skills such as memory, executive function, processing speed and attention, among others. There are several commercially available cognitive training programs. Find one that you enjoy and are therefore more likely to engage in regularly. Beware of programs that claim scientific validity but are not associated with published, peer-reviewed studies.

individuals. Participants in the memory training group showed improved memory and those in the InSight group showed improved processing speed and memory. Both interventions were also associated with improved self-ratings of cognitive function and quality of life.

The effect sizes for both the Lumosity and InSight study were moderate, meaning that not everyone improved. It is unknown which of these programs is better for cancer-related cognitive effects because the two have not been directly compared. Additionally, it is unknown if another cognitive training program would show equal or better results. Lumosity provides exercises in multiple cognitive domains including executive function and memory. InSight focuses on processing speed but InSight is part of a more comprehensive suite of cognitive exercises provided by Posit Science called BrainHQ. Both Lumosity and BrainHQ are subscription-based services with relatively similar fees ($7-$8/month for a yearly subscription). Both services offer free trials and Lumosity has a 30-day money back guarantee. These programs are available online meaning that you will need an internet-connected computer to use them. You can also use them on an iPhone or iPad with the BrainHQ app or the Lumosity Brain Trainer app.

CogMed (http://www.cogmed.com/) is another computerized cognitive training program. Several research studies support its effectiveness in non-cancer populations [159,160] but it has not been tested in cancer survivors to date. Lumosity and Posit Science are available for independent, home-based cognitive exercise while CogMed is available only through qualified professionals. It is not currently known which is better - doing cognitive training on your own or with a clinician's supervision. It may depend on individual preferences and cognitive strengths and weaknesses. For example, someone who is struggling with self-motivation and follow-through may have better outcome working with a clinician than working on his/her own.

It is important to find a cognitive training program that you enjoy and that works for you. Lumosity, Posit Science and CogMed have the most research support thus far. However, there are several other cognitive training programs you can choose from. You can find them online by searching for "brain training". Many cognitive training programs claim to have scientific validation but you should look carefully at the references provided. Proper clinical trials are published in medical or scientific journals. An easy test of validity is to search for the title of the scientific reference in PubMed (http://www.ncbi.nlm.nih.gov/pubmed).

As with physical exercise, irregular or inconsistent cognitive training may not result in much improvement and thus it is critical to engage in your cognitive exercises on a regular schedule. There currently are no interventions available that provide immediate results or "cure" cognitive difficulties following cancer. A commitment to regular, consistent effort will provide the best results. Unfortunately, the research thus far is unclear regarding how long or how often one should engage in cognitive exercises. Most successful clinical trials of cognitive training have involved multiple training sessions that were distributed regularly over many weeks or months. One study suggested that as little as 10 hours of training can have lasting benefit [156]. However, this study involved healthy adults who did not have existing cognitive problems and therefore individuals who are experiencing cognitive difficulties may require longer training.

The stability of cognitive training benefits over time, after training has ended, is also not well know. Only a few studies have examined long-term retention of training benefits but suggest that these benefits may continue up to five years later in healthy adults [156,161]. Cognitive training effects do seem to show dose-dependence. In other words, more training may mean more benefit [151]. Additionally, completing "booster sessions" may result in increased benefit. For example, one study showed that healthy adults who completed a four hour booster session 11 months after completing their original training program showed the largest improvements in cognitive function [156].

If you are engaging in cognitive training on your own, try starting out with four to five, 30-60 minute sessions per week for at least six weeks. If you observe that the training is helpful, you can continue on with the same schedule or stop the training and do a booster session (four to five 30-60 minute sessions per week for 2-3 weeks) every six to 12 months. If the cognitive training does not seem to be helping, try extending the training to 12 weeks. At that time, you can decide whether to continue on the same schedule, move into booster mode, try a different cognitive training program (perhaps one with clinician guidance) or try alternate strategies for coping with cognitive effects.

Cognitive exercise does not have to be computerized. There are board games such as chess and also books that include puzzles and brain teasers. The goal is to identify activities that challenge you and result in learning something new. If a cognitive exercise is too easy, your brain will not be stimulated enough. If it is too difficult, you will be less likely to stick with the exercise. It can be tricky but not impossible to adjust the difficulty of non-computerized exercises. For example, if you enjoy chess, you can study and learn new chess strategies. You could try to find opponents who are slightly better than you to play against. If you like reading, you can choose books that contain dense or unfamiliar content. Discussing books with others, such as in a book club, can also be very stimulating and challenging for the brain.

However, difficulty level is one area where computerized exercises have a distinct advantage. Computers can implement sophisticated algorithms that increase or decrease the difficulty level so that there is a balance between success and challenge. This automation can make computerized cognitive exercises more convenient. Another advantage of computer-based exercises is that you can track your progress over time. Most cognitive training programs record performance metrics such as accuracy and reaction time that you can access. These programs often provide a comparison of your performance with that of other individuals your age. Some programs even include cognitive tests that you can routinely take to see how your various cognitive skills are progressing.

This brings up one of the main criticisms of computerized cognitive training. Some believe that these exercises simply improve one's performance on cognitive tests but have no effect on, or transfer to real-world tasks. Many computerized cognitive training exercises are similar to the standardized neuropsychological tests that are used to measure training outcome. This remains an area of ongoing debate in the field of cognitive training. Some of the controversy seems to stem from the fact that earlier research studies simply did not include measures of real-world outcomes and therefore the transfer of skills could not be adequately evaluated. More recent studies, like those conducted with cancer survivors as described above, provide evidence that cognitive training can transfer skills to real-life behaviors. Specifically, participants in these studies showed significant improvement on self-ratings of cognitive skills and quality of life. This suggests that the participants observed positive effects of the cognitive training program during everyday life demands.

Also, these studies indicated that the computerized cognitive training programs improved cognitive skills that were not actually trained. For example, the InSight Posit Science processing speed program improved processing speed but also improved memory. The Lumosity program focused on executive function and was associated with improved executive function but also increased memory. Participants in these studies also reported decreased depression, anxiety and fatigue [157,158]. One study of older, non-cancer adults with insomnia demonstrated that computerized cognitive training improved sleep quality including how quickly patients went to sleep and how much time they spent asleep [162]. These findings suggest that cognitive training can potentially improve a variety of problematic symptoms in addition to cognitive performance. This makes sense given that cognitive training targets brain biology, which underlies psychiatric symptoms such as depression, anxiety and sleep disruption as well as cognitive skills.

There are no known side effects to cognitive training. You may experience some frustration during difficult tasks but this should be temporary. If you become overly frustrated, take a break from the cognitive exercise and try it again later. It is probably best to practice a variety of mental tasks and cognitive exercises so that certain skills do not become out of balance. For example, if you practice only memory skills, other skills like processing speed, attention or executive function might be neglected.

Active Journaling

Another way to exercise your mind and reduce stress is through active journaling. A study founded by Dr. David Snowdon at the University of Minnesota has followed 678 Catholic nuns since 1986 in order to better understand some of the environmental factors that might contribute to Alzheimer's disease. Study researchers examined samples of the nuns' autobiographical writings and discovered that higher "idea density" was associated with increased protection of the brain from age-related cognitive decline [163,164]. Idea density refers to the average number of ideas expressed within a certain number of words. An idea-dense statement provides the reader with a lot of relevant information in a very concise, efficient manner.

You can practice developing idea-dense language skills by writing in a journal. This exercise can also help you practice other skills including thinking, memory and organization. However, this is more than just writing down what happened to you during the day. *Active* journaling requires you to discuss what you thought and felt about various events and why. When you actively journal, you are striving to describe the meaning of your activities and experiences. What inspires you and why? What interactions did you have with others and what did they mean to you? What new things did you learn? What do you think about certain events, ideas or people and why?

Get a journal or notebook or use a word processing program on the computer. There are also several tablet-based and smartphone apps for journaling. If you don't like writing or typing, use the voice recognition feature on your tablet, smartphone or computer. There are also specific computer programs that can convert your voice to text.

Think about an experience you had, a news story you heard, a conversation you had or something you did and write about why it was important to you, what it meant to you and/or what you learned from it. The important aspect of this exercise is to analyze, interpret, think about and express your thoughts, feelings and ideas. In addition to content, your grammar, spelling and writing are also important. Emphasizing all of these components will help you exercise your language and communication skills. Journaling also helps with your memory because you are required to recall events, thoughts and feelings that occurred during the day.

Here is an example entry: "Today I went to museum with Sarah and there was a painting I particularly liked. It was by Georges Braque. I had not heard of him before so I read some of the captions near the painting. I learned that he was a contemporary of Picasso and they introduced a new form of painting that included a collage technique. They introduced painted words and imitations of wood or marble in their paintings, sometimes mixing sawdust or sand into the paint. Their work blurred the lines between painting and sculpture.

I have never really been a big fan of Picasso's work because it mostly makes me feel unsettled. It seems that his human figures especially are distorted or disfigured. I now have a better understanding of his technique. He was trying to show his figures as they look from a variety of different perspectives – the perspectives you might get from having a more 3-dimensional form. Depending on our perspective, certain objects from certain viewpoints might actually look somewhat

Ideas..
Thoughts..
Interests..

Insights...
Feelings..

Goals...

What did I
learn today?

Writing in a journal can be an excellent way to exercise your brain by practicing your memory, thinking, organization and communication skills. It is important to analyze, ponder and expand upon your thoughts, ideas and feelings rather than simply recording them.

distorted. Braque's paintings involve a lot of musical expression that I identify with. This painting that I especially liked seemed to show the music exploding from the main form in the painting. The colors were rather muted – mostly browns and golds – but the form of the painting conveyed the passion of the music and so I understood why people thought these works were more similar to sculptures."

In this example, the writer documented what she learned, thought and felt about something she observed in her environment. The entry is relatively brief which can help focus and organize thoughts. You should try to keep your individual entries to two pages or less. This will help you practice being efficient, or more "idea dense" in your communication.

Here is another example entry: "I had an appointment with my oncologist today and she told me that I need to be more active. I am a bit overweight and tend to sit too much. She told me that this is not good for my recovery and can actually increase my risk for cancer relapse. I know that she is right but it is difficult to get out there and do something. I feel very lazy and unmotivated. Sometimes when I eat things I shouldn't eat and don't exercise, I think, "Oh well, what's the point?" and then I just eat more and sit around more. It's very self-defeating. However, I talked to my husband and we are making a goal to walk for at least 45 minutes every other day. It will help to have his support so that I don't feel so alone in this effort."

This entry is obviously simpler than the first example but it can be effective and helpful to write some of your feelings about various things and also record your goals and achievements. You should read over your previous journal entries on a regular basis. This will help you remember things and will also let you see how you progress over time with various thoughts, feelings and achievements.

Journal entries do not have to be limited to factual life occurrences. Creative writing such as poetry or short stories can be very effective mental exercise. You do not need any previous creative writing experience or training. You do not ever have to show your writing to anyone so feel free to write whatever you want. Other ideas for creative writing include taking an event from your past that you wished had gone differently and writing about how you wanted it to happen. You could write about an event that takes place in your future. How do you envision your life one year from now or 10 years from now? Try to write in your journal regularly (for example, once per day or 4 times per week). Find a schedule that you can consistently stick with.

Cognitive Reserve

Unlike physical exercise where changes such as weight loss and increased stamina are readily observed, you may not notice changes due to cognitive exercise. Even standardized neuropsychological tests are not always sensitive to changes due to cognitive exercises. However, cognitive exercise is believed to increase **cognitive reserve**, which is not easily measured. Cognitive reserve refers to neural resources that increase the brain's efficiency and resilience. Cognitive reserve is like having a savings account. The more money in your savings account, the better protected you are from the effects of economic recession or unemployment. The more cognitive reserve you have, the better protected you are from the effects of brain injury, illness and aging. Research shows that cancer survivors with higher cognitive reserve (i.e. patients who are more mentally active) have less cognitive difficulties [27,105].

Cognitive reserve is something that can always be increased throughout the lifespan via simple behavioral changes [165]. Cognitive training provides a structured way to exercise your brain that automatically increases the difficulty as you improve. However, any activity that enriches your environment and stimulates your mind will potentially increase cognitive reserve. Activities such as crossword puzzles, visiting museums, reading, watching educational programs, participating in social discussions/groups/clubs, playing board games or chess, playing a musical instrument, reading the newspaper or magazines, doing original art or craft work or taking a course, among other things can help keep your mind active. The key components for activities that increase cognitive reserve are engaging in them regularly and consistently and using them to challenge and stimulate your mind. For example, reading alone may not be enough to increase cognitive reserve. You must study, ponder, discuss and/or reflect (verbally or in writing) on what you are reading. Reading about topics that are novel or challenging for you will be more effective.

Prevention

Could cognitive training done prior to and/or during cancer treatment *prevent* cognitive decline? As described above, cognitive training can help prevent age-related cognitive decline in healthy adults. Also, a history of regular mental activity has been shown to help protect against cognitive difficulties following chemotherapy. However, the effectiveness of cognitive training as a preventative intervention is currently unknown. There may be periods during disease and treatment course when cognitive training is more or less effective.

For example, one study randomized 96 patients undergoing adjuvant chemotherapy to one of two cognitive training programs (computerized or in-person) or a control (no training) group. They found that were no intervention effects [166]. However, the participants in this study were only two months, on average, off-therapy and thus the study results may have been confounded by the control group's natural brain recovery. In general, rehabilitative cognitive training is believed to be more effective if initiated after the patient has stabilized medically and neurologically [167]. Previous studies suggest that intensive cognitive therapy during acute periods of recovery provide no benefit beyond what is associated with spontaneous recovery and can even lead to poorer outcomes in some cases [167]. Poorer outcome likely stems from pushing the brain too fast, too soon while it is trying to recover from injury. However, this may only apply to more severe injuries such as those associated with brain tumor or radiation necrosis.

Research suggests that patients with breast cancer continue to show cognitive changes within the first year off-therapy [21,22] and therefore cognitive training might be more optimally implemented after this period, when the brain has stabilized. In fact, cognitive training has been found to be highly effective in the chronic recovery period, even when implemented multiple years after the initial injury in non-cancer populations [168]. Thus far, studies demonstrating benefit of cognitive training or rehabilitation in breast cancer survivors have excluded patients who were not at least one year off chemotherapy and radiation [143,157,158].

There is currently no available method of predicting which cognitive difficulties a certain patient will have so it is not possible to know which cognitive skills to target for prevention. A preventative cognitive training program could simply include a wide variety of cognitive skills or just those that are most commonly affected by cancer and cancer treatments. These approaches could potentially increase cognitive reserve. However, it is possible that preventative cognitive training would need to be fundamentally different from current cognitive training methods in some presently unknown manner in order to be effective. For example, prevention training might need to involve different types of exercises or different algorithms for adapting difficulty level compared to regular cognitive training.

Despite the uncertainty, mental activity does seem to be associated with increased neuroprotection as well as reduced depression, anxiety and fatigue. Therefore, there may be some benefit from engaging in cognitive exercise before and during cancer treatments. Less formal mental activities such as journaling, reading, chess or artwork may be more feasible and tolerable before and during treatment. It may be easier to focus on and follow through with more structured and intensive cognitive training programs after treatment.

The timing of more structured, intensive cognitive training will likely also depend on the type of cancer treatment involved. Based on the research thus far, breast cancer survivors have been shown to benefit from cognitive training starting 6-12 months after chemotherapy and radiation have ended. Many patients receive hormonal blockade therapy for several years and therefore it is unclear when formal cognitive training would be of most benefit for them. However, previous studies of cognitive training in cancer survivors have included patients who were still actively receiving hormone therapy [157,158]. Therefore, these patients might be able to begin cognitive training at anytime. For patients with brain tumor, cognitive rehabilitation has not begun until patients were medically stable for at least six months.

In summary, cognitive exercise may help improve cognitive skills and/or protect the brain against further decline. Cognitive exercise should be regular, consistent and involve activities that are challenging and ideally result in new learning. There are several computerized cognitive exercise programs that have preliminary research support for use in cancer survivors. Other activities such as active journaling can also be effective. It is important to find an activity or activities that you enjoy and will engage in regularly. There currently are no established guidelines for how much or how often to engage in cognitive exercise. A schedule of 30-60 minutes, four to five times per week is generally consistent with many research studies. However, finding a schedule that you can reliably stick with is the most important consideration. It is unknown whether structured cognitive training can help prevent cognitive difficulties if done before or during cancer treatment. It may be more difficult to focus on a cognitive training program during this time resulting in increased frustration and lower benefit. However, regular mental activity is generally beneficial for all individuals and therefore informal mental activities could help protect against cognitive decline.

Chapter 6: Compensatory Strategies

In addition to practicing and improving cognitive skills and increasing cognitive reserve, you may also need ways to compensate for certain cognitive difficulties so that you can perform daily tasks with success. When the brain is injured, it often loses the ability to automatically solve problems and therefore it requires some re-training in strategic approaches. These strategies might range from simple scripts for talking oneself through the steps of a particular task to the use of assistive technology for cuing, initiation and reminding.

External Aids

One of the most effective and essential strategies for improving cognitive performance is the use of external aids to remind, organize, cue and track. These external aids may take many forms depending on your personal preferences, resources and technological expertise. Using a notebook or day planner to keep track of appointments, to-do lists, goals and other important information can help with memory and organization. Technology such as smartphones and pagers provide more sophisticated memory aids. If you have a smartphone, try using the calendar and alert/reminder functions to help you with memory tasks. Most smartphones include built-in calendar and reminder applications, but you can also purchase specialized applications for your smartphone such that were designed for people with cognitive difficulties. Calendar and reminder applications have alert functions where you can set an alarm (audible signal and/or vibrating signal) that will tell you about an upcoming appointment or task deadline. You can typically set these alarms to occur minutes, hours or days before the appointment or deadline.

Additionally, most smartphones now have voice recognition software so that you can simply say a command (e.g. "Remind me to call Susan at 3 o'clock today") rather than having to type on the small keyboard. Smartphone applications not only help you with memory tasks but can also assist with navigation, managing your finances, organizing medications, tracking diet and exercise and many other daily activities. You can even obtain applications ("apps") that allow you to do your cognitive exercises using your smartphone.

Use a smartphone or other similar device, a day planner or notebook to manage your schedule, keep track of to-do lists and deadlines. While a day planner or notebook might initially be easier and less intimidating to use, a smartphone or other electronic device has the distinct advantage of being able to alert you to upcoming events and deadlines. Be sure to set aside time in your schedule for cognitive exercises, physical activity and relaxation training.

However, the data plans required by smartphones can be expensive. If you do not wish to purchase such a data plan, you can also try using a mobile device. This is a small, easy to use, handheld device that has calendar and reminder applications as well as voice recognition but does not require a data plan. Like a phone, you can carry it with you everywhere you go in order to keep track of your schedule, to-do list and other helpful information. There are several portable devices available that can provide electronic assistance similar to a smartphone.

Learning how to use these technological devices can be intimidating if you are unused to them. Take this as a challenge that will help exercise your brain! Do not be afraid to experiment with the device in order to figure it out. There are free videos online that show you the basic functions of a smartphone, for example. Ask a friend or family member who is technologically savvy to teach you how to use your device. An occupational therapist might also be able to provide you with some individual training if necessary.

Routines

Oftentimes, cognitive performance, especially memory, can be improved by establishing a set routine. This helps to minimize how much you have to remember. It is best to schedule tasks and appointments on the same days and times every week whenever possible. Keep important items such as your keys, purse, wallet, etc. in the same exact location everyday. Create a specific place for these items that is easily visible in your home or office. Associate difficult to remember tasks with other tasks. For example, always take your medication at dinnertime or right before watching the morning news. Complete tasks in the same order every time; for example, (1) brush teeth, (2) take medication, (3) eat breakfast, (4) review daily schedule, (5) check email, etc. When you establish routines in this manner, they will become habits and your brain will start to implement them automatically. Routines work best for tasks that you do frequently. For procedures or tasks that you must perform infrequently, write down step-by-step instructions – like a recipe – and keep these notes in a central location such as a specific desk drawer, in your smartphone or on your computer. Include pictures when possible.

Establishing set routines can also help you form healthy habits. As noted in Chapter 5, there are many activities that can help improve your cognitive function. However, you will need to do these regularly in order for them to be optimally effective. This requires getting into the habit of doing them. In addition to appointments, it is helpful to specifically schedule activities such as cognitive exercises, journaling, relaxation and physical exercise. You can enter these activities in your external device (e.g. smartphone) calendar and have the schedule repeat every day or several times per week. This will help set aside time for these goals, make them routine and remind you to do them.

Self-Talk

Self-talk is a cognitive strategy that aims to improve attention, memory and executive function through verbal statements that prompt, guide and maintain behaviors. This self-talk procedure works by providing cues and structure for controlling behaviors. Self-instruction was initially developed as an intervention for impulsive children but has since been widely applied to assist both children and adults with improving cognitive function. It has been shown to be highly effective in improving cognitive performance following brain injuries [169].

To apply the self-talk strategy, you simply say aloud or silently the steps that you must take to accomplish a particular goal or task. Here are some example scripts for self-talk to help with certain skills.

Planning

Every Sunday evening, review your schedule and/or to do list for the upcoming week. As you review it, say aloud the following questions:

"What am I supposed to be doing?" State what appointments you have scheduled.

"What do I need to do to prepare for these events/appointments?" State what preparations you need to make.

"What obstacles might I encounter and how can I prepare for or avoid them?" State the obstacles you might encounter.

"Is there anything I forgot?"

Repeat this script every morning with respect to your daily schedule. If you are using assistive technology (e.g. smartphone), make sure all your appointments and to-do's are entered into your device and that reminder alerts for each of them are set.

Attention

During tasks, say aloud the following:

"What should I be doing right now?" State what you should be doing.

"What do I need to do next?" State what you should do next.

Problem Solving

Use the following script for various goal-oriented or problem based tasks:

"Stop and think."

"What am I doing?" State the main task.

"How should I do this?" State the main steps for accomplishing the task.

Execute the task.

"What am I doing right now?" State what you are doing.

"What do I need to do next?" State what step comes next.

"Am I doing what I planned to do?" State whether or not you are following your plan.

"How is this working out?" State your progress and any problems or difficulties.

"Is there a better way to do this?" State your evaluation of the plan and progress and any alternate ideas or approaches you think of.

Memory Strategies

One of the most effective strategies for improving memory and learning is repetition. In the past, you may have required only a few exposures to information before you remembered it. If you are currently struggling with memory, you will likely need to practice and repeat the information more often in order to keep it stored. Making notes, creating routines and setting reminders can reduce the amount of information that you must keep track of and therefore reduce the chances that you will forget something important.

When trying to learn new information, use both verbal and visual cues when possible. Make sketches or diagrams or find pictures that help summarize the information you need to remember. For example, this book includes illustrations

whenever possible in order to aid in the understanding and recall of the information it contains. Visual cues can often communicate information much more concisely than verbal cues. The combination of both visual and verbal cues will help strengthen your recall of the information.

Many cancer survivors have difficulty with verbal or auditory memory – recalling information that one has heard. This most often occurs when someone is telling you something or during a social conversation. Some individuals with verbal memory problems lose track of the conversation, repeat themselves or forget what the other person was saying. These are all examples of verbal memory difficulty.

One strategy for improving your verbal recall is called active listening. When you are talking with someone else, you must try to keep what the person is saying in your memory as well as what you want to say back. This working memory task can be very difficult. Reflective listening can help because it forces you to pay more attention to what the other person is saying, which is usually the harder thing to remember. If you can remember what the other person is saying, this will usually cue your memory about what you wanted to say as well. When someone is talking to you, your goal is to periodically paraphrase (repeat using your own words) what they have just said. For example:

Dr. Smith: "So your test results are very positive. I'm glad to see that you have been following the guidelines I gave you during our last visit. To maintain these changes, I would like you to take this medication 2 times a day for 2 weeks and also I want you to exercise at least 3 times per week for 30 minutes."

Patient: "So it sounds like I'm doing better but I still need to take this medication twice a day for 2 weeks and workout for 30 minutes 3 times a week?"

Dr. Smith: "That's correct."

Active listening also ensures that you understand what has been said to you. You can seek clarification if necessary. Pause before you jump in and begin talking. This will give you time to think about what has been said and what you are going to say.

Here are some examples of reflective listening statements:

"It sounds like...."

"What I hear you saying..."

"It seems as if...."

"I get the sense that...."

"It feels as though...."

You will likely remember what people have said to you more easily since you will have to concentrate on their words in order to be able to paraphrase them correctly. It is also a good idea to take notes during important conversations such as when you meet with your physician.

Paraphrasing or summarizing other types of information can also aid memory. For example, when you read, pause periodically to paraphrase what you have just read either aloud, silently or in writing. This helps to repeat and reinforce the information but also to condense it into a smaller, more manageable form. The "In summary..." sections at the end of each chapter in this book as well as the entire Chapter 9 provide examples of how to paraphrase key concepts into concise summaries.

Situational Control

Not all cognitive difficulties are due to cancer or cancer treatments. Some cognitive difficulties are the result of normal mistakes that everyone experiences from time to time and are more likely in certain situations. Factors such as stress, pain, hunger, lack of sleep, time pressure and lack of preparation can increase the likelihood of cognitive difficulties for *anyone*. Many of these factors can be anticipated and prevented in order to reduce the chance of cognitive failures.

You should be sure to address issues such as depression, sleep disruption, fatigue and pain with your doctor to reduce their influence on your cognitive functions (see Chapter 7). Try to avoid engaging in complex cognitive tasks during times of the day when you are more likely to be tired or fatigued. Take regular rest breaks throughout the day. Make sure to give yourself plenty of time to accomplish your goals or tasks. Try to reduce distractions or find a quiet area to work when possible. Focus on one thing at a time and then move on to the next item. Slow down and take additional time to prepare for your goals. When a cognitive mistake occurs, try to think of what was happening right before. Were you stressed? Tired? Hungry? In pain? Did you try to do something at the last minute? Were there too many distractions? There are likely several factors that you have control over and can therefore modify to increase your chances of success.

Workplace Accommodations

Cognitive difficulties can make returning to work a significant challenge. Many cancer survivors find that they are unable to return to work at the same level or same number of hours as before their diagnosis. Survivors report that work tasks tend to require more effort and/or the use of alternative strategies

[170]. Returning back to work too quickly may actually worsen cognitive difficulties by pushing the brain too fast, too soon while it is trying to recover from injury. Starting back to work at part-time and gradually increasing to full-time is often helpful. Cancer and chemotherapy-related cognitive difficulties may qualify for workplace accommodations under the Americans with Disabilities Act (ADA, http://www.ada.gov). Talk with your human resources representative before returning to work to ensure that you understand your rights and benefits.

Recommendations for specific workplace accommodations often require a neuropsychological evaluation (see Chapter 4) and/or documentation from your physician. Accommodations can include things like extended time for assignments and learning of new tasks, allowance for rest breaks, relocation/redesign of workspace, modified work schedule and job restructuring, among others. Specific accommodations will likely be based on your individual cognitive strengths and weaknesses. It is recommended that you discuss potential accommodations with your neuropsychologist.

Talk with your supervisor regarding your cognitive difficulties before you return to work. You may need to help educate him or her regarding the cognitive effects of cancer and its treatments. Ask your supervisor for his or her ideas and suggestions for helping make your return successful and be prepared to provide your own suggestions. Your neuropsychologist may be able to help advocate for accommodations and/or advise regarding appropriate accommodations by speaking with your employer. You can find further information regarding reasonable accommodation examples and the procedure for requesting them from your employer here:

http://www.eeoc.gov/policy/docs/accommodation.html

In summary, there are several strategies you can adopt that will help you compensate for cognitive difficulties. These include using external aids such as a notebook, day planner or electronic device to keep track of important information. You can establish routines to make certain actions more automatic and reduce the number of tasks you must actively remember. Self-talk can help with various executive functions including planning and problem solving. Use repetition, paraphrasing, note taking and visual cues to aid memory and learning. Keep in mind that some cognitive failures are just normal mistakes that can sometimes be prevented by reducing situation factors such as stress, pain, distractions and procrastination. Finally, if you are employed, there are certain accommodations that may help increase your success in the workplace. Talk with your human resources manager and supervisor as well as your neuropsychologist and/or physician regarding appropriate workplace accommodations.

Chapter 7: Stress Management

Psychiatric symptoms including anxiety, depression and sleep disruption are very common following cancer. Depression is characterized by sadness, loss of interest, and feelings of hopelessness, helplessness or worthlessness. Anxiety involves feelings of worry, fear or nervousness. Sleep disruption refers to difficulty falling or staying asleep. Insomnia is a type of sleep disruption common in cancer survivors [171].

These symptoms are normal responses to the stress of being ill, which often includes having one's life disrupted, experiencing a change in cognitive function, dealing with physical pain, concern regarding financial resources and fear of relapse, among other stressors. These symptoms are often the result of a complex interaction of biological and psychosocial factors. Cancer/chemotherapy can result in damage to brain regions like the prefrontal cortex that are important for regulating emotion, causing increased vulnerability to psychiatric difficulties. Psychiatric symptoms increase cognitive difficulties, which then in turn increase psychiatric distress.

When the brain is affected by an illness or injury, it sometimes loses its ability to correctly judge what is threatening or not threatening. It therefore switches to a survival mode where it interprets most things as threatening – it tends to be hypersensitive and overreact. Think about how you might feel if your arm were broken. You would likely be much more protective of it than you normally would to prevent further injury. This is what often happens within the brain as well. It has been injured and becomes more protective of itself and the rest of your body.

If your brain correctly perceives a threat when there really is one or perceives no threat when there really isn't one, everything is good. However, if it does not perceive a threat when there really is a threat, this could be very bad. This is how your brain interprets the world when it has been injured. In order to avoid a serious mistake, such as perceiving no

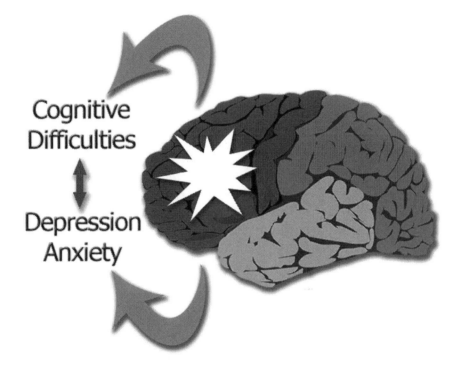

Cancer and its treatments are associated with injury to brain regions like the prefrontal cortex. This injury can result in cognitive difficulties but also increased vulnerability to psychiatric distress including depression and anxiety. Furthermore, concern over cognitive difficulties can increase psychiatric symptoms and psychiatric symptoms tend to worsen cognitive difficulties. Therefore, stress management is an essential strategy for improving cognitive function.

threat when there really is a threat, your brain overcompensates or becomes overly cautious by interpreting many things as threats. As a result, you may feel like little things bother you that didn't before or that you overreact and have less tolerance for loud or crowded places, driving in traffic, talking to people, etc. You might feel anxious, fearful and nervous. This is a normal response to being injured – you feel more vulnerable to even the mildest potential dangers.

Although this is a protective mechanism, it can obviously interfere with your daily functioning and can become chronic and maladaptive if left unchecked. Fortunately, you can learn to reduce and control this protective response through relaxation exercises. This chapter provides several such exercises that you can try. It is very important for your cognitive recovery that you try to practice relaxation and stress management daily. Chronic stress can worsen cognitive difficulties and can also negatively impact your physical health. For example, research suggests that cancer survivors with symptoms of depression have double the risk for mortality [172].

Patients experience varying levels of emotional trauma following their illness. Some patients experience mild symptoms that may remit over time while others demonstrate significant difficulties such as major depression or post-traumatic stress disorder (PTSD) that require clinical intervention. Treatments for psychiatric symptoms include psychotherapy and/or medication. Talk to your health care provider if you are having symptoms of depression or anxiety and are unsure if you require clinical intervention or not.

Stressors are events that result in a stress response. They can be internal or external. Internal stressors include thoughts, emotions and memories. External stressors are typically things that happen in the environment such as a traffic accident, an argument with a family member or an injury. Whether or not a particular stressor results in a stress response depends on the individual's subjective interpretation of it and his/her previous experiences, current psychological and physical health and personal history.

The body responds to stressors by engaging in a "fight or flight" reaction. The brain perceives the stressor as a threat, triggering a release of hormones including adrenaline and cortisol, which result in several physiologic changes including increased heart rate, blood pressure and glucose release. Non-critical systems such as digestion are suppressed to divert resources towards mechanisms that will promote survival such as brain and muscles for quick thinking and action. After the stressor has passed or resolved, the body returns to normal.

However, patients with cancer often experience chronic stress responses due to physical and emotional consequences of the illness. Cancer is often a major stressor in and of itself but can also make an individual more vulnerable to other stressors due to brain and other physiologic changes that make the person less resilient to stress. Prolonged stress response exhausts the body's resources and its resistance to stress. Continued stress is detrimental to nearly all physiological systems, increasing the risk for heart disease, immune dysfunction, sleep disturbance, digestive problems, obesity and other difficulties. Chronic stress tends to be associated with increased levels of hormones and inflammatory molecules that can cause further damage to brain structures.

Relaxation Exercise

During prolonged stress response, the body loses its natural ability to self-regulate and return to homeostasis. Therefore, conscious relaxation efforts are required to reduce the detrimental effects of chronic stress on physical and psychological health. Individuals have a surprising amount of conscious control over the stress response although this often requires consistent practice for optimal effectiveness. There is a large body of research that supports the use of relaxation techniques in reducing the effects of chronic stress and increasing physical and psychological health. Relaxation techniques have measurable, positive effects on brain function [173,174] and can help with improving sleep. There are many different relaxation techniques. This chapter describes three options: autogenics, progressive muscle relaxation and guided imagery. Practice at least one of these or some other relaxation exercise every day for 20-30 minutes.

Autogenics

This stress management technique involves progressively relaxing various body areas such as arms, legs, etc. It is implemented through meditative self-instruction statements such as "my legs feel warm and heavy" that are repeated several times. Your mind has a great deal of control over your physiological responses and with practice, you can improve your ability to elicit a relaxed state through these simple self-instruction methods. When starting out, it is easier to have a recorded script that you can follow.

Progressive Muscle Relaxation (PMR)

As described above, the stress response involves activation of muscle groups in preparation for fight or flight. During chronic stress, muscle tension often persists. PMR is a relaxation technique that involves alternating between tensing and relaxing various major muscle groups throughout the body. PMR is believed to reduce anxiety by increasing awareness regarding muscle tension and developing control over the release of this tension. By focusing on muscle tension and relaxation, the mind is also given a break from distressing thoughts and feelings. You can find audio recordings that will guide you through a PMR exercise. You can find various PMR recordings and scripts online if you prefer to try different voices and music. PMR will involve flexing muscles and then quickly and completely releasing them. You should flex muscles only about 30%. If you have any muscle pain or injured areas, do not flex that muscle group but simply focus on relaxing it.

Guided Imagery

You can achieve a relaxed state when you imagine all the details of a safe, comfortable place, such as a beach or a garden – a "getaway" or "happy place." You can use an instructor, recording or written scripts to help you through this process.

Using all of your senses, your body seems to respond as though what you are imagining is real. For example, imagine that you are holding a lemon. Think in great detail about the smell, the color and the texture of the peel. Then see yourself taking a bite of the lemon and feel the juice squirting into your mouth. Many people salivate when they do this.

Imagery techniques have been repeatedly shown to enhance skill learning and performance in athletes, surgeons and musicians [175]. In these studies, simply imagining the proper actions improved the actual performance of them. Other studies show that imagery can accelerate rehabilitation of physical function after brain injury [175]. These examples demonstrate how your body can respond to what you are only imagining.

It is often best to practice guided imagery for relaxation using a pre-recorded script while sitting or lying in a quiet place. As you develop your own imagined getaway, you can call upon it quickly at any time throughout the day. For example, when feeling anxious, take a deep breath and visualize your getaway. Imagery is also very useful for dealing with physical pain or relieving feelings of boredom. You can find guided imagery recordings from several sources.

These are just a few examples of relaxation techniques. As with the other interventions described in this book, it is important that you find a relaxation technique you like and that works for you. Other examples include mindfulness meditation and cognitive restructuring. Activities such as Tai chi and Hatha yoga are also good choices for stress management.

In summary, stress management is critical for improving cognitive function and preventing further cognitive decline. It is very important that you address any psychiatric symptoms such as depression, anxiety or sleep disruption. These symptoms may require clinical intervention such as medication and/or psychotherapy. It is recommended that you engage in relaxation exercises 20-30 minutes everyday to help manage stress symptoms. There are several relaxation techniques you can try and it is important to find one that works for you so that you will engage in it regularly.

Chapter 8: Physical Exercise

Regular physical activity has been shown not only to decrease stress but also to improve and protect cognitive function [176,177]. In fact, studies have shown significant improvements in cognitive and brain function in as little as one month following a regular exercise program [178]. In one study, 358 cancer survivors were randomly assigned to a four-week yoga intervention (two, 75 minute sessions per week) or to a control group that did not receive the yoga sessions. Compared to the control group, survivors who completed the yoga program demonstrated significantly improved memory function [179]. The yoga intervention involved breathing exercises, gentle Hatha and Restorative yoga postures and meditation [179-181]. Another study examined 408 patients newly diagnosed with breast, genitourinary, lung, gastrointestinal, hematologic, gynecologic or head/neck cancer. Patients who exercised during and/or after treatment demonstrated improved health and memory and reduced fatigue compared to patients who did not exercise [182].

Physical exercise can also help reduce symptoms of anxiety, depression, fatigue and sleep disruption. In two additional studies of yoga, 410 cancer survivors were randomly assigned to the yoga intervention or a control group. Survivors who completed the yoga sessions demonstrated significantly improved quality of life, circadian rhythms and mood as well as decreased fatigue, sleep medication use and anxiety compared to those assigned to the control group [180,181].

Aerobic exercise has been shown to significantly increase the number of new neurons in the hippocampus, even after one day [183]. Exercise increases the levels of certain neurotransmitters (chemicals) in the brain that promote cognitive function [184]. Exercise also increases the expression of certain neuro-protective genes in the brain [184] and reduces inflammation [185]. Physical activity decreases the risk for Alzheimer's disease and can slow age-related cognitive decline [184,186]. Exercise helps with maintaining a healthy weight, which can decrease the risk for certain cancers and cancer recurrence [187].

Moderate activity
(60% maximum HR)
150 mins per week

or vigorous activity
(70% maximum HR)
120 mins per week

220 - age = maximum HR

Regular physical activity can improve brain function and protect the brain from further decline. Activity that increases your heart rate (HR) to at 60-70% of your maximum HR is recommended. Calculate your maximum HR by subtracting your current age from 220.

To improve brain function, it is recommended that you engage in moderate intensity exercise at least 150 minutes per week or vigorous exercise at least 120 minutes per week (e.g. 20 minutes [178]. For example, you could exercise at moderate intensity for at least 30 minutes on five or more days per week, at vigorous intensity for at least 20 minutes on three or more days a week, or some combination of the two. Moderate exercise is defined as activity that increases your heart rate to 60% of your maximum. Vigorous exercise increases your heart rate to 70% of your maximum.

To calculate your maximum heart rate, subtract your current age from 220 (220 – your age). For example, a 55 year old person's maximum heart rate is 165. Then multiple your maximum heart rate by 60% to determine your moderate intensity heart rate and by 70% to determine your vigorous intensity heart rate. A 55 year old would need to increase his or her heart rate to at least 99 beats per minute for moderate activity and to approximately 115 beats per minute for vigorous activity. You can use a heart rate monitor during your exercise session to track your heart rate and keep it within the target zone or simply pause your activity every 10 or 15 minutes and take your pulse from your wrist. Take your pulse for 30 seconds and multiple it by 2.

Moderate intensity exercises include walking at a pace of approximately three miles per hour (mph), cycling on flat terrain at five to nine mph, yoga, dancing, weight lifting, or using a stationary bike, stair climber or rowing machine at a moderate effort setting. Examples of vigorous intensity exercises include jogging, running, speed walking, walking uphill, circuit weight training, boxing or using exercise machines at a vigorous effort setting. More examples can be found at the Centers for Disease Control and Prevention website (http://www.cdc.gov/physicalactivity/). To avoid injury, you may need to gradually work up to moderate/vigorous intensity exercise if you have been sedentary for an extended time.

As with cognitive skills, external aids can be very useful in helping you achieve your goals for physical activity. Research shows that individuals who consistently engage in self-monitoring show increased fitness and weight loss compared to those who do not consistently self-monitor [188-191]. Using a notebook or other paper diary to record and monitor physical activity as well as food intake can be very effective in enhancing adherence to healthy behaviors. Technology can make this self-monitoring task easier. There are several fitness tracking websites available that allow you to sync your activity with a smartphone other mobile device.

Pedometers and activity monitors are small electronic devices that help track health behaviors. Pedometers track the number of steps taken. Activity monitors track your activity level, sleep, diet and calories burned. They provide motivational cues, reinforcement and reminders. These devices sync with your smartphone, tablet and/or computer and allow you to track your progress over time. There are several different affordable activity monitors available that can be worn on the wrist or hip and have various features for tracking and encouraging activity. Many smartphones and the new "smart watches" have activity monitoring capabilities.

Social support can be an essential motivating factor for engaging in physical activity [192]. Exercising with another person or group of people is often more rewarding than doing it alone and the social interaction is good for your brain function. Involving others in your physical activity goals increases your accountability – it's often more difficult to find an excuse not to exercise when someone else is expecting you at the gym or meeting you for a walk. Participating in group exercise classes is another way to get increased social support for your physical activity goals and can also help you expand your social network. Most of the self-monitoring aids such as the websites and devices described above provide you the option of sharing your progress with others. Some friendly competition along with mutual encouragement can be very motivating.

Find a schedule that you can consistently stick with and choose activities that you enjoy so that you are more likely to continue doing them. You do not have to run marathons or do Olympic lifting - just focus on elevating your heart rate and oxygen consumption. Activities such as walking and yoga can be excellent options. Even simple changes to your daily routine can make a difference. Try parking farther away from your destination so that you walk a greater distance. Is your destination close enough that you could walk there instead of driving? Take the stairs instead of the elevator or escalator. Go on a short walk after dinner. If you have physical or medical limitations, you can still be active. Research shows that even doing non-aerobic stretching and toning can result in some brain function improvement [178]. However, moderate intensity exercise is recommended for lasting brain health and to protect against health-related risks such as cancer relapse. You may want to consider consulting with your physician, a physical therapist or personal trainer to determine the best fitness program for you.

Both physical and cognitive exercises increase the number of neurons in the hippocampus. The effect on hippocampal neurogenesis is unique for each exercise type. Physical exercise results in an increased number of new neurons. Unfortunately, around 50% of these new cells die within a few weeks, having never reached full maturity or becoming connected with other neurons [183]. However, many of these neurons can potentially be saved with cognitive training, particularly if the training is challenging and results in learning. These rescued neurons remain in the hippocampus and form functional connections within brain networks [183]. Therefore, the combination of physical and cognitive exercise may result in increased cognitive benefit compared to physical or cognitive training alone.

In summary, regular physical activity is important for cognitive function as well as general health and longevity. It is recommended that you engage in moderate intensity exercise at least 150 minutes per week, vigorous activity 120 minutes per week or some combination of the two. Find activities and a schedule that you can reliably engage in. Focus on elevating your heart rate and oxygen consumption. Keep track of your physical activity and diet using a paper diary or electronic device.

Chapter 9: Wrapping Up

Cognitive difficulties are common after cancer and its treatments. The possible reasons for these cognitive changes include suppression of neural progenitor cells, damage to DNA, disruption of immune system function and genetic vulnerabilities, among others. These mechanisms ultimately result in brain injury that reduces the brain's ability to function effectively and efficiently. Brain changes show improvement in some patients but not in others and some patients demonstrate increased cognitive problems over time. Therefore, it is an important part of your ongoing cancer survivorship plan to monitor and address cognitive difficulties. The first step often involves obtaining a neuropsychological evaluation to determine your cognitive strengths and weaknesses and formulate an individual treatment plan. You might also want to talk to your doctor about potential medications that could help with cognitive difficulties. Additionally, seek treatment for depression, anxiety and sleep disruption (e.g. insomnia) if necessary as these symptoms can worsen cognitive difficulties.

In addition, you can engage in a comprehensive program of independent interventions that may help improve cognitive function and/or prevent ongoing cognitive decline. This program includes cognitive exercise, physical activity, stress management and compensatory strategies. Cognitive exercise involves computerized games, active journaling or other mentally challenging activities. Physical exercise involves activities that elevate your heart rate to 60-70% of its maximum, 120-150 minutes per week. Maximum heart rate is determined by subtracting your current age from 220. Stress management includes relaxation exercises 20-30 minutes per day, everyday. Compensatory strategies include using a smartphone or other similar device to track appointments, tasks and deadlines and to set reminders, using active listening, routines, repetition and paraphrasing to aid memory, using self-talk to help with executive functions, and obtaining workplace accommodations as needed. These strategies can help you to accomplish daily tasks and minimize cognitive failures.

Two final recommendations for dealing with cognitive effects of cancer and its treatments include (1) utilize your social support network and (2) stay informed. Educate your family and friends regarding cognition and cancer and solicit their assistance in adhering to your intervention program. Consider participating in a cancer survivorship group to share your experiences dealing with cognitive effects and to learn what others have found helpful. See if there are research studies going on in your area that you could participate in. Being a research volunteer not only tends to give you access to breaking research findings but also can help you feel like you are contributing to the search for a solution. You can find open research studies from several sources including Army of Women (http://www.armyofwomen.org), ClinicalTrials.gov (http://www.clinicaltrials.gov) and Research Match (https://www.researchmatch.org).

There also are several resources available to help you stay informed regarding the latest research findings in the field of cognition and cancer (as well as any other research topic). PubMed (http://www.ncbi.nlm.nih.gov/pubmed) provides many research articles in full text for free. In fact, all federally funded research studies are required to be submitted to PubMed Central, the National Institutes of Health free full text archive of scientific journal articles. Additionally, many cancer centers, research labs and other groups of interest are active on social media such as Facebook and Twitter.

Cognitive difficulties can be very challenging and distressing. It may seem cruelly ironic that the treatments helping you to survive may be contributing to your inability to remember, pay attention or think of the word you want to say. Surviving cancer is an ongoing process that does not end after treatment is over. Be patient with yourself. Remember that some mistakes are normal. Don't give up. Your brain is biologically programmed to adapt, improve and become more efficient with consistent effort. Have courage. You have just taken another important step in your recovery by learning more regarding how to cope with cognitive difficulties.

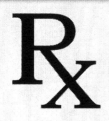

1. Neuropsychological evaluation

2. Cognitive exercises 30-60 mins per day, 4-5 days per week

3. Physical activity that elevates the heart rate to 60-70% of maximum 120-150 mins per week

4. Relaxation exercises 20-30 mins per day, everyday

5. Compensatory strategies to help with daily tasks

6. Address any symptoms of anxiety, depression, fatigue or sleep disruption

Although currently there is no specific cure for cancer-related cognitive difficulties, there are several interventions that may help improve cognitive function and/or prevent further decline.

About the Author

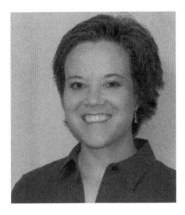

Dr. Shelli Kesler is a clinical neuropsychologist and cognitive neuroscientist with extensive experience in the evaluation and treatment of individuals with brain injuries. She is an Associate Professor of Neuro-oncology at the University of Texas MD Anderson Cancer Center. Her laboratory specializes in research that focuses on the cognitive effects of cancer and chemotherapy. She was a 2008 recipient of the National Institutes of Health New Innovator Award for her work in this area.

Glossary

Allele: An alternate form of the same gene, one member of a pair of genes.

Alzheimer's disease: a brain disorder that typically affects older adults characterized by progressively worsening cognitive function including decline in memory, executive function, language and other cognitive functions such that independent living skills are often significantly compromised.

Anemia: a lack of healthy red blood cells resulting in reduced oxygen supply to body tissues.

Anxiety: A psychiatric state or condition characterized by worry, nervousness or fear.

Astrocyte: A type of cell whose function in the brain is to support neurons and perform repair and clean up.

Attention: The ability to focus or concentrate on specific information.

Blood-brain barrier: A cellular and molecular barrier that restricts access to the brain.

Brain network: A group of brain regions that work together to support particular cognitive processes.

Cell differentiation: A process during which a cell reaches maturity and becomes the type of cell it is programmed to become.

Cell proliferation: Cell growth or division that results in new cells.

Cerebellum: A brain structure located at the bottom of the brain that is important for motor coordination as well as higher-order cognitive skills including speech and emotion processing.

Chemo brain: A common term used to describe cognitive problems such as difficulties with memory or thinking following chemotherapy treatment.

Choline: A chemical or metabolite in the brain that is believed to be a marker of neuron density and/or rate of cell membrane turnover. Choline is also a precursor of the neurotransmitter acetylcholine which is essential for several cognitive functions.

CNS: Central nervous system. Part of the nervous system consisting of the brain and spinal cord that is responsible for information processing and coordination of responses.

Cognition: A set of mental process stemming from brain function. Examples include memory, attention, executive function, reasoning, problem solving and understanding language.

Cognitive flexibility: A core executive function characterized by the ability to generate multiple alternative solutions to problems and switch fluidly between thoughts or actions.

Cognitive rehabilitation: A behavioral or psychological treatment for cognitive difficulties that typically aims to restore cognitive functioning and/or help patients learn to compensate for cognitive difficulties.

Cognitive reserve: Protection of the brain from injury or illness stemming from mental and/or physical activity.

Cognitive training: A program of mental activity that typically involves repeated practice of cognitive skills where the practice is adaptive, or becomes more difficult as one progresses.

Cranium: The space inside the skull that is occupied by the brain.

Cytokine: A molecule involved in regulating immune system function and responses.

Dementia: A brain disorder characterized by progressive cognitive decline.

Depression: A psychiatric state or condition characterized by sadness, loss of interest, feelings of hopelessness, helplessness or worthlessness.

DNA: Deoxyribonucleic acid. A molecule that contains the set of genetic instructions necessary for the development and function of living organisms.

Executive function: A set of mental processes important for preparing complex behaviors and adapting to the environment.

Gray matter: A type of brain tissue consisting of neuron bodies involved in information processing.

Hippocampus: A structure located in the medial temporal lobe of the brain that is critical for learning and memory. The hippocampus is one of only two sites of ongoing neurogenesis in the adult brain.

Intracranial pressure: pressure inside the cranium that is exerted on the brain.

Memory: A mental process concerned with the storage and retrieval of information.

Myelin: An insulating material that forms around the axon of a neuron and facilitates rapid communication between neurons.

Myo-inositol: A chemical or metabolite in the brain that is considered a marker of glial cell function. Glial cells play a role in inflammation.

N-acetylaspartate: A chemical or metabolite in the brain that is believed to be a marker of neuron health or number.

Neural compensation: A neuroplasticity process during which the brain attempts to counteract dysfunction by recruiting additional brain resources such as activating alternate regions or networks to help support cognitive response.

Neural progenitor cells: Neural stem and precursor cells that generate new neurons and other brain cells within the hippocampus.

Neurogenesis: The creation of new neurons in the hippocampus.

Neuroimaging: A method of viewing and measuring various aspects of the brain including volume, white matter integrity, functional activity and metabolism, among others.

Neuroinflammation: Inflammation within the brain.

Neuron: A brain cell that processes and transmits information. A neuron is comprised of a body, axon and dendrites.

Neuroplasticity: The ability of the brain to reorganize itself to support new learning, repair, compensation and adaptation.

Neuropsychology: The study of brain-behavior relationships.

Neuropsychological evaluation: A process during which the brain is assessed for strengths and weaknesses using standardized tests in combination with review of a patient's history and symptoms.

Neurotransmitter: A chemical that transmits signals between neurons.

Oligodendrocyte: A type of brain cell involved in the formation of myelin.

Oxidative stress: An increase in the byproducts of oxygen metabolism resulting in an environment that is toxic to cells.

Pathological: Caused by a disease.

Physical exercise: Activity of the body that increases heart rate and oxygen consumption.

Placebo: An inert or non-therapeutic treatment provided as a control to compare with an active treatment to determine treatment effectiveness.

Prefrontal cortex: A region of the brain responsible for executive function, language, memory, emotion and other complex cognitive skills.

Processing speed: The speed at which the brain is able to process information.

Radiation necrosis: Degradation of brain tissue following radiotherapy, typically to the head or neck.

Response inhibition: A core executive function characterized by the suppression of actions that interfere with goal-directed behavior.

Self-renewal: The ability of stem cells to replicate themselves.

Systemic chemotherapy: Chemotherapy that is typically delivered intravenously (i.e. IV) or orally (e.g. pills) rather than directly into the CNS. Many systemic chemotherapies do not actively cross the blood-brain barrier.

White matter: A type of brain tissue consisting of myelinated axons of neurons involved in the communication of information between brain regions.

Working memory: A core executive function characterized by the short-term maintenance and manipulation of information.

References

1. Wefel JS, Witgert ME, Meyers CA. Neuropsychological sequelae of non-central nervous system cancer and cancer therapy. Neuropsychol Rev 2008;18:121-31. doi: 10.1007/s11065-008-9058-x
2. Schagen SB, Muller MJ, Boogerd W, Mellenbergh GJ, van Dam FS. Change in cognitive function after chemotherapy: a prospective longitudinal study in breast cancer patients. Journal of the National Cancer Institute 2006;98:1742-5. doi: 10.1093/jnci/djj470
3. Stewart A, Collins B, Mackenzie J, Tomiak E, Verma S, Bielajew C. The cognitive effects of adjuvant chemotherapy in early stage breast cancer: a prospective study. Psychooncology 2008;17:122-30. doi: 10.1002/pon.1210
4. Phillips KM, Jim HS, Small BJ, Laronga C, Andrykowski MA, Jacobsen PB. Cognitive functioning after cancer treatment: a 3-year longitudinal comparison of breast cancer survivors treated with chemotherapy or radiation and noncancer controls. Cancer 2012;118:1925-32. doi: 10.1002/cncr.26432
5. Scherling C, Collins B, Mackenzie J, Bielajew C, Smith A. Prechemotherapy differences in response inhibition in breast cancer patients compared to controls: a functional magnetic resonance imaging study. J Clin Exp Neuropsychol 2012;34:543-60. doi: 10.1080/13803395.2012.666227
6. Scherling C, Collins B, Mackenzie J, Bielajew C, Smith A. Pre-chemotherapy differences in visuospatial working memory in breast cancer patients compared to controls: an FMRI study. Front Hum Neurosci 2011;5:122. doi: 10.3389/fnhum.2011.00122
7. Schonberg T, Pianka P, Hendler T, Pasternak O, Assaf Y. Characterization of displaced white matter by brain tumors using combined DTI and fMRI. NeuroImage 2006;30:1100-11.
8. Wei CW, Guo G, Mikulis DJ. Tumor effects on cerebral white matter as characterized by diffusion tensor tractography. The Canadian journal of neurological sciences Le journal canadien des sciences neurologiques 2007;34:62-8.
9. Zeller B, Tamnes CK, Kanellopoulos A, et al. Reduced Neuroanatomic Volumes in Long-Term Survivors of Childhood Acute Lymphoblastic Leukemia. J Clin Oncol 2013;31:2078-85. doi: 10.1200/JCO.2012.47.4031
10. Koppelmans V, Groot MD, de Ruiter MB, et al. Global and focal white matter integrity in breast cancer survivors 20 years after adjuvant chemotherapy. Hum Brain Mapp 2012. doi: 10.1002/hbm.22221
11. Koppelmans V, de Ruiter MB, van der Lijn F, et al. Global and focal brain volume in long-term breast cancer survivors exposed to adjuvant chemotherapy. Breast Cancer Res Treat 2012;132:1099-106. doi: 10.1007/s10549-011-1888-1

12. Bergouignan L, Lefranc JP, Chupin M, Morel N, Spano JP, Fossati P. Breast cancer affects both the hippocampus volume and the episodic autobiographical memory retrieval. PLoS ONE 2011;6:e25349. doi: 10.1371/journal.pone.0025349

13. Kesler S, Janelsins M, Koovakkattu D, et al. Reduced hippocampal volume and verbal memory performance associated with interleukin-6 and tumor necrosis factor-alpha levels in chemotherapy-treated breast cancer survivors. Brain Behav Immun 2013;30 Suppl:S109-16. doi: 10.1016/j.bbi.2012.05.017

14. Inagaki M, Yoshikawa E, Matsuoka Y, et al. Smaller regional volumes of brain gray and white matter demonstrated in breast cancer survivors exposed to adjuvant chemotherapy. Cancer 2007;109:146-56.

15. McDonald BC, Conroy SK, Ahles TA, West JD, Saykin AJ. Gray matter reduction associated with systemic chemotherapy for breast cancer: a prospective MRI study. Breast Cancer Research and Treatment 2010;123:819-28. doi: 10.1007/s10549-010-1088-4

16. McDonald BC, Conroy SK, Smith DJ, West JD, Saykin AJ. Frontal gray matter reduction after breast cancer chemotherapy and association with executive symptoms: a replication and extension study. Brain Behav Immun 2013;30 Suppl:S117-25. doi: 10.1016/j.bbi.2012.05.007

17. Cimprich B, Reuter-Lorenz P, Nelson J, et al. Prechemotherapy alterations in brain function in women with breast cancer. J Clin Exp Neuropsychol 2010;32:324-31. doi: 913518343 [pii]10.1080/13803390903032537

18. Hosseini SM, Koovakkattu D, Kesler SR. Altered small-world properties of gray matter networks in breast cancer. BMC Neurol 2012;12:28. doi: 10.1186/1471-2377-12-28

19. Kesler SR, Bennett FC, Mahaffey ML, Spiegel D. Regional brain activation during verbal declarative memory in metastatic breast cancer. Clin Cancer Res 2009;15:6665-73. doi: 10.1158/1078-0432.CCR-09-1227

20. Silverman DH, Dy CJ, Castellon SA, et al. Altered frontocortical, cerebellar, and basal ganglia activity in adjuvant-treated breast cancer survivors 5-10 years after chemotherapy. Breast Cancer Res Treat 2007;103:303-11. doi: 10.1007/s10549-006-9380-z

21. Correa DD, Ahles TA. Neurocognitive changes in cancer survivors. Cancer J 2008;14:396-400. doi: 10.1097/PPO.0b013e31818d876900130404-200811000-00008 [pii]

22. Wefel JS, Saleeba AK, Buzdar AU, Meyers CA. Acute and late onset cognitive dysfunction associated with chemotherapy in women with breast cancer. Cancer 2010;116:3348-56. doi: 10.1002/cncr.25098

23. Reuter-Lorenz PA, Cimprich B. Cognitive function and breast cancer: promise and potential insights from functional brain imaging. Breast Cancer Res Treat 2013;137:33-43. doi: 10.1007/s10549-012-2266-3

24. Ferguson RJ, McDonald BC, Saykin AJ, Ahles TA. Brain structure and function differences in monozygotic twins: possible effects of breast cancer chemotherapy. J Clin Oncol 2007;25:3866-70. doi: 25/25/3866 [pii]10.1200/JCO.2007.10.8639

25. McDonald BC, Conroy SK, Ahles TA, West JD, Saykin AJ. Alterations in Brain Activation During Working Memory Processing Associated With Breast Cancer and Treatment: A Prospective Functional Magnetic Resonance Imaging Study. J Clin Oncol 2012;30:2500-8. doi: 10.1200/JCO.2011.38.5674

26. de Ruiter MB, Reneman L, Boogerd W, et al. Cerebral hyporesponsiveness and cognitive impairment 10 years after chemotherapy for breast cancer. Hum Brain Mapp 2011;32:1206-19. doi: 10.1002/hbm.21102

27. Kesler SR, Kent JS, O'Hara R. Prefrontal cortex and executive function impairments in primary breast cancer. Archives of neurology 2011;68:1447-53. doi: 10.1001/archneurol.2011.245

28. Bruno J, Hosseini SM, Kesler S. Altered resting state functional brain network topology in chemotherapy-treated breast cancer survivors. Neurobiol Dis 2012;48:329-38. doi: 10.1016/j.nbd.2012.07.009

29. Heimans JJ, Reijneveld JC. Factors affecting the cerebral network in brain tumor patients. J Neurooncol 2012;108:231-7. doi: 10.1007/s11060-012-0814-7

30. Bartolomei F, Bosma I, Klein M, et al. Disturbed functional connectivity in brain tumour patients: evaluation by graph analysis of synchronization matrices. Clin Neurophysiol 2006;117:2039-49. doi: 10.1016/j.clinph.2006.05.018

31. Hsieh TC, Wu YC, Yen KY, Chen SW, Kao CH. Early Changes in Brain FDG Metabolism during Anticancer Therapy in Patients with Pharyngeal Cancer. Journal of neuroimaging : official journal of the American Society of Neuroimaging 2013. doi: 10.1111/jon.12006

32. Chao HH, Uchio E, Zhang S, et al. Effects of androgen deprivation on brain function in prostate cancer patients - a prospective observational cohort analysis. BMC cancer 2012;12:371. doi: 10.1186/1471-2407-12-371

33. Janelsins MC, Kohli S, Mohile SG, Usuki K, Ahles TA, Morrow GR. An update on cancer- and chemotherapy-related cognitive dysfunction: current status. Seminars in oncology 2011;38:431-8. doi: 10.1053/j.seminoncol.2011.03.014

34. Wefel JS, Schagen SB. Chemotherapy-related cognitive dysfunction. Current neurology and neuroscience reports 2012;12:267-75. doi: 10.1007/s11910-012-0264-9

35. Ahles TA, Saykin AJ, McDonald BC, et al. Cognitive function in breast cancer patients prior to adjuvant treatment. Breast Cancer Res Treat 2008;110:143-52. doi: 10.1007/s10549-007-9686-5

36. Ganz PA, Bower JE, Kwan L, et al. Does tumor necrosis factor-alpha (TNF-α) play a role in post-chemotherapy cerebral dysfunction? Brain, Behavior, and Immunity 2013;30:S99-S108. doi: 10.1016/j.bbi.2012.07.015

37. Whiteside TL. Immune suppression in cancer: Effects on immune cells, mechanisms and future therapeutic intervention. Seminars in Cancer Biology 2006;16:3-15.

38. Seruga B, Zhang H, Bernstein LJ, Tannock IF. Cytokines and their relationship to the symptoms and outcome of cancer. Nat Rev Cancer 2008;8:887-99. doi: nrc2507 [pii]10.1038/nrc2507

39. Vardy JL, Booth C, Pond GR, et al. Cytokine levels in patients (pts) with colorectal cancer and breast cancer and their relationship to fatigue and cognitive function. J Clin Oncol (Meeting Abstracts) 2007;25:9070.

40. Talacchi A, Santini B, Savazzi S, Gerosa M. Cognitive effects of tumour and surgical treatment in glioma patients. J Neurooncol 2011;103:541-9. doi: 10.1007/s11060-010-0417-0

41. Satoer D, Vork J, Visch-Brink E, Smits M, Dirven C, Vincent A. Cognitive functioning early after surgery of gliomas in eloquent areas. J Neurosurg 2012;117:831-8. doi: 10.3171/2012.7.JNS12263

42. Teixidor P, Gatignol P, Leroy M, Masuet-Aumatell C, Capelle L, Duffau H. Assessment of verbal working memory before and after surgery for low-grade glioma. J Neurooncol 2007;81:305-13. doi: 10.1007/s11060-006-9233-y

43. Schilder CM, Seynaeve C, Linn SC, et al. Cognitive functioning of postmenopausal breast cancer patients before adjuvant systemic therapy, and its association with medical and psychological factors. Crit Rev Oncol Hematol 2010;76:133-41. doi: 10.1016/j.critrevonc.2009.11.001

44. Debess J, Riis JO, Pedersen L, Ewertz M. Cognitive function and quality of life after surgery for early breast cancer in North Jutland, Denmark. Acta Oncol 2009;48:532-40. doi: 10.1080/02841860802600755

45. Chen ML, Miaskowski C, Liu LN, Chen SC. Changes in perceived attentional function in women following breast cancer surgery. Breast Cancer Res Treat 2012;131:599-606. doi: 10.1007/s10549-011-1760-3

46. Hanning CD. Postoperative cognitive dysfunction. British journal of anaesthesia 2005;95:82-7. doi: 10.1093/bja/aei062

47. Newman S, Stygall J, Hirani S, Shaefi S, Maze M. Postoperative cognitive dysfunction after noncardiac surgery: a systematic review. Anesthesiology 2007;106:572-90.

48. Caza N, Taha R, Qi Y, Blaise G. The effects of surgery and anesthesia on memory and cognition. Prog Brain Res 2008;169:409-22. doi: 10.1016/S0079-6123(07)00026-X

49. Johnson T, Monk T, Rasmussen LS, et al. Postoperative cognitive dysfunction in middle-aged patients. Anesthesiology 2002;96:1351-7.

50. Vacas S, Degos V, Feng X, Maze M. The neuroinflammatory response of postoperative cognitive decline. Br Med Bull 2013;106:161-78. doi: 10.1093/bmb/ldt006

51. Wang Y, Sands LP, Vaurio L, Mullen EA, Leung JM. The effects of postoperative pain and its management on postoperative cognitive dysfunction. Am J Geriatr Psychiatry 2007;15:50-9. doi: 10.1097/01.JGP.0000229792.31009.da

52. Deeken JF, Loscher W. The blood-brain barrier and cancer: transporters, treatment, and Trojan horses. Clin Cancer Res 2007;13:1663-74. doi: 10.1158/1078-0432.CCR-06-2854

53. Ahles TA, Saykin AJ. Candidate mechanisms for chemotherapy-induced cognitive changes. Nat Rev Cancer 2007;7:192-201. doi: nrc2073 [pii]10.1038/nrc2073

54.   Dietrich J, Han R, Yang Y, Mayer-Proschel M, Noble M. CNS progenitor cells and oligodendrocytes are targets of chemotherapeutic agents in vitro and in vivo. J Biol 2006;5:22. doi: jbiol50 [pii]10.1186/jbiol50

55.   Hyrien O, Dietrich J, Noble M. Mathematical and experimental approaches to identify and predict the effects of chemotherapy on neuroglial precursors. Cancer Res 2010;70:10051-9. doi: 10.1158/0008-5472.CAN-10-1400

56.   Dietrich J. Chemotherapy associated central nervous system damage. Advances in experimental medicine and biology 2010;678:77-85.

57.   Wigmore PM, Mustafa S, El-Beltagy M, Lyons L, Umka J, Bennett G. Effects of 5-FU. Adv Exp Med Biol 2010;678:157-64.

58.   Seigers R, Schagen SB, Coppens CM, et al. Methotrexate decreases hippocampal cell proliferation and induces memory deficits in rats. Behav Brain Res 2009;201:279-84. doi: S0166-4328(09)00142-9 [pii]10.1016/j.bbr.2009.02.025

59.   Seigers R, Schagen SB, Beerling W, et al. Long-lasting suppression of hippocampal cell proliferation and impaired cognitive performance by methotrexate in the rat. Behav Brain Res 2008;186:168-75. doi: S0166-4328(07)00403-2 [pii]10.1016/j.bbr.2007.08.004

60.   Winocur G, Vardy J, Binns MA, Kerr L, Tannock I. The effects of the anti-cancer drugs, methotrexate and 5-fluorouracil, on cognitive function in mice. Pharmacology, biochemistry, and behavior 2006;85:66-75.

61.   Han R, Yang YM, Dietrich J, Luebke A, Mayer-Proschel M, Noble M. Systemic 5-fluorouracil treatment causes a syndrome of delayed myelin destruction in the central nervous system. Journal of Biology 2008;7:12. doi: 10.1186/jbiol69

62.   Janelsins MC, Mustian KM, Palesh OG, et al. Differential expression of cytokines in breast cancer patients receiving different chemotherapies: implications for cognitive impairment research. Supportive Care in Cancer 2012;20:831-9. doi: 10.1007/s00520-011-1158-0

63.   Pusztai L, Mendoza TR, Reuben JM, et al. Changes in plasma levels of inflammatory cytokines in response to paclitaxel chemotherapy. Cytokine 2004;25:94-102.

64.   Tsavaris N, Kosmas C, Vadiaka M, Kanelopoulos P, Boulamatsis D. Immune changes in patients with advanced breast cancer undergoing chemotherapy with taxanes. British journal of cancer 2002;87:21-7. doi: 10.1038/sj.bjc.6600347

65.   Collado-Hidalgo A, Bower JE, Ganz PA, Cole SW, Irwin MR. Inflammatory biomarkers for persistent fatigue in breast cancer survivors. Clin Cancer Res 2006;12:2759-66. doi: 10.1158/1078-0432.CCR-05-2398

66.   Wilson CJ, Finch CE, Cohen HJ. Cytokines and cognition--the case for a head-to-toe inflammatory paradigm. Journal of the American Geriatrics Society 2002;50:2041-56.

67.   Wong ML, Bongiorno PB, al-Shekhlee A, Esposito A, Khatri P, Licinio J. IL-1 beta, IL-1 receptor type I and iNOS gene expression in rat brain vasculature and perivascular areas. Neuroreport 1996;7:2445-8.

68.   Konsman JP, Vigues S, Mackerlova L, Bristow A, Blomqvist A. Rat brain vascular distribution of interleukin-1 type-1 receptor immunoreactivity: relationship to patterns of inducible cyclooxygenase expression by peripheral inflammatory stimuli. J Comp Neurol 2004;472:113-29. doi: 10.1002/cne.20052

69.   Anthony DC, Bolton SJ, Fearn S, Perry VH. Age-related effects of interleukin-1 beta on polymorphonuclear neutrophil-dependent increases in blood-brain barrier permeability in rats. Brain 1997;120 (Pt 3):435-44.

70.   Lynch MA. Age-related neuroinflammatory changes negatively impact on neuronal function. Front Aging Neurosci 2010;1:6. doi: 10.3389/neuro.24.006.2009

71.   Aluise CD, Miriyala S, Noel T, et al. 2-Mercaptoethane sulfonate prevents doxorubicin-induced plasma protein oxidation and TNF-alpha release: implications for the reactive oxygen species-mediated mechanisms of chemobrain. Free radical biology & medicine 2011;50:1630-8. doi: 10.1016/j.freeradbiomed.2011.03.009

72.   Joshi G, Aluise CD, Cole MP, et al. Alterations in brain antioxidant enzymes and redox proteomic identification of oxidized brain proteins induced by the anti-cancer drug adriamycin: implications for oxidative stress-mediated chemobrain. Neuroscience 2010;166:796-807. doi: 10.1016/j.neuroscience.2010.01.021

73.   Joshi G, Hardas S, Sultana R, St Clair DK, Vore M, Butterfield DA. Glutathione elevation by gamma-glutamyl cysteine ethyl ester as a potential therapeutic strategy for preventing oxidative stress in brain mediated by in vivo administration of adriamycin: Implication for chemobrain. J Neurosci Res 2007;85:497-503. doi: 10.1002/jnr.21158

74.   Tangpong J, Cole MP, Sultana R, et al. Adriamycin-mediated nitration of manganese superoxide dismutase in the central nervous system: insight into the mechanism of chemobrain. J Neurochem 2007;100:191-201. doi: JNC4179 [pii]10.1111/j.1471-4159.2006.04179.x

75.   Tangpong J, Cole MP, Sultana R, et al. Adriamycin-induced, TNF-alpha-mediated central nervous system toxicity. Neurobiology of disease 2006;23:127-39. doi: 10.1016/j.nbd.2006.02.013

76.   Chen Y, Jungsuwadee P, Vore M, Butterfield DA, St Clair DK. Collateral damage in cancer chemotherapy: oxidative stress in nontargeted tissues. Molecular interventions 2007;7:147-56. doi: 10.1124/mi.7.3.6

77.   Conroy SK, McDonald BC, Smith DJ, et al. Alterations in brain structure and function in breast cancer survivors: effect of post-chemotherapy interval and relation to oxidative DNA damage. Breast Cancer Res Treat 2013;137:493-502. doi: 10.1007/s10549-012-2385-x

78.   Ahles TA. Brain vulnerability to chemotherapy toxicities. Psychooncology 2012;21:1141-8. doi: 10.1002/pon.3196

79.   Deprez S, Amant F, Smeets A, et al. Longitudinal Assessment of Chemotherapy-Induced Structural Changes in Cerebral White Matter and Its Correlation With Impaired Cognitive Functioning. J Clin Oncol 2012;30:274-81. doi: 10.1200/JCO.2011.36.8571

80.   de Ruiter MB, Reneman L, Boogerd W, et al. Late effects of high-dose adjuvant chemotherapy on white and gray matter in breast cancer survivors: converging results from multimodal magnetic resonance imaging. Hum Brain Mapp 2012;33:2971-83. doi: 10.1002/hbm.21422

81.   Raichle ME. The restless brain. Brain connectivity 2011;1:3-12. doi: 10.1089/brain.2011.0019

82.   Damoiseaux JS. Resting-state fMRI as a biomarker for Alzheimer's disease? Alzheimer's research & therapy 2012;4:8. doi: 10.1186/alzrt106

83.   Kesler SR, Wefel JS, Hosseini SM, Cheung M, Watson CL, Hoeft F. Default mode network connectivity distinguishes chemotherapy-treated breast cancer survivors from controls. Proceedings of the National Academy of Sciences of the United States of America 2013;110:11600-5. doi: 10.1073/pnas.1214551110

84.   Kesler SR, Watson C, Koovakkattu D, et al. Elevated prefrontal myo-inositol and choline following breast cancer chemotherapy. Brain Imaging Behav 2013;7:501-10. doi: 10.1007/s11682-013-9228-1

85.   Bozgeyik Z, Burakgazi G, Sen Y, Ogur E. Age-related metabolic changes in the corpus callosum: assessment with MR spectroscopy. Diagnostic and interventional radiology 2008;14:173-6.

86.   Wang T, Xiao S, Li X, et al. Using proton magnetic resonance spectroscopy to identify mild cognitive impairment. International psychogeriatrics / IPA 2011:1-9. doi: 10.1017/S1041610211000962

87.   Heck JE, Albert SM, Franco R, Gorin SS. Patterns of dementia diagnosis in surveillance, epidemiology, and end results breast cancer survivors who use chemotherapy. Journal of the American Geriatrics Society 2008;56:1687-92. doi: 10.1111/j.1532-5415.2008.01848.x

88.   Du XL, Xia R, Hardy D. Relationship between chemotherapy use and cognitive impairments in older women with breast cancer: findings from a large population-based cohort. Am J Clin Oncol 2010;33:533-43. doi: 10.1097/COC.0b013e3181b9cf1b

89.   Kesler SR, Watson CL, Blayney DW. Brain network alterations and vulnerability to simulated neurodegeneration in breast cancer. Neurobiology of Aging 2015. doi: 10.1016/j.neurobiolaging.2015.04.015

90.   Winick N. Neurocognitive outcome in survivors of pediatric cancer. Current opinion in pediatrics 2011;23:27-33. doi: 10.1097/MOP.0b013e32834255e9

91.   Levin VA, Bidaut L, Hou P, et al. Randomized double-blind placebo-controlled trial of bevacizumab therapy for radiation necrosis of the central nervous system. Int J Radiat Oncol Biol Phys 2011;79:1487-95. doi: 10.1016/j.ijrobp.2009.12.061

92.   Monje ML, Palmer T. Radiation injury and neurogenesis. Current opinion in neurology 2003;16:129-34.

93.   Monje ML, Mizumatsu S, Fike JR, Palmer TD. Irradiation induces neural precursor-cell dysfunction. Nat Med 2002;8:955-62. doi: 10.1038/nm749nm749 [pii]

94.   Monje M. Cranial radiation therapy and damage to hippocampal neurogenesis. Dev Disabil Res Rev 2008;14:238-42. doi: 10.1002/ddrr.26

95. Greene-Schloesser D, Robbins ME, Peiffer AM, Shaw EG, Wheeler KT, Chan MD. Radiation-induced brain injury: A review. Frontiers in oncology 2012;2:73. doi: 10.3389/fonc.2012.00073

96. Daams M, Schuitema I, van Dijk BW, et al. Long-term effects of cranial irradiation and intrathecal chemotherapy in treatment of childhood leukemia: a MEG study of power spectrum and correlated cognitive dysfunction. BMC Neurol 2012;12:84. doi: 10.1186/1471-2377-12-84

97. Donovan KA, Small BJ, Andrykowski MA, Schmitt FA, Munster P, Jacobsen PB. Cognitive functioning after adjuvant chemotherapy and/or radiotherapy for early-stage breast carcinoma. Cancer 2005;104:2499-507. doi: 10.1002/cncr.21482

98. Jim HS, Donovan KA, Small BJ, Andrykowski MA, Munster PN, Jacobsen PB. Cognitive functioning in breast cancer survivors: a controlled comparison. Cancer 2009;115:1776-83. doi: 10.1002/cncr.24192

99. Formenti SC, Demaria S. Systemic effects of local radiotherapy. The Lancet Oncology 2009;10:718-26. doi: 10.1016/s1470-2045(09)70082-8

100. Collins B, Mackenzie J, Stewart A, Bielajew C, Verma S. Cognitive effects of chemotherapy in post-menopausal breast cancer patients 1 year after treatment. Psychooncology 2009;18:134-43. doi: 10.1002/pon.1379

101. Castellon SA, Ganz PA, Bower JE, Petersen L, Abraham L, Greendale GA. Neurocognitive performance in breast cancer survivors exposed to adjuvant chemotherapy and tamoxifen. J Clin Exp Neuropsychol 2004;26:955-69.

102. Schilder CM, Seynaeve C, Beex LV, et al. Effects of tamoxifen and exemestane on cognitive functioning of postmenopausal patients with breast cancer: results from the neuropsychological side study of the tamoxifen and exemestane adjuvant multinational trial. J Clin Oncol 2010;28:1294-300. doi: JCO.2008.21.3553 [pii]10.1200/JCO.2008.21.3553

103. Palmer JL, Trotter T, Joy AA, Carlson LE. Cognitive effects of Tamoxifen in pre-menopausal women with breast cancer compared to healthy controls. J Cancer Surviv 2008;2:275-82. doi: 10.1007/s11764-008-0070-1

104. Shilling V, Jenkins V, Fallowfield L, Howell T. The effects of hormone therapy on cognition in breast cancer. J Steroid Biochem Mol Biol 2003;86:405-12.

105. Ahles TA, Saykin AJ, McDonald BC, et al. Longitudinal Assessment of Cognitive Changes Associated With Adjuvant Treatment for Breast Cancer: Impact of Age and Cognitive Reserve. Journal of Clinical Oncology 2010;28:4434-40. doi: 10.1200/jco.2009.27.0827

106. Ahles TA, Saykin AJ, Furstenberg CT, et al. Neuropsychologic impact of standard-dose systemic chemotherapy in long-term survivors of breast cancer and lymphoma. J Clin Oncol 2002;20:485-93.

107. Eberling JL, Wu C, Tong-Turnbeaugh R, Jagust WJ. Estrogen- and tamoxifen-associated effects on brain structure and function. NeuroImage 2004;21:364-71. doi: S1053811903005457 [pii]

108. Ernst T, Chang L, Cooray D, et al. The effects of tamoxifen and estrogen on brain metabolism in elderly women. J Natl Cancer Inst 2002;94:592-7.

109.   Cherrier MM, Aubin S, Higano CS. Cognitive and mood changes in men undergoing intermittent combined androgen blockade for non-metastatic prostate cancer. Psychooncology 2009;18:237-47. doi: 10.1002/pon.1401

110.   Cherrier MM, Borghesani PR, Shelton AL, Higano CS. Changes in neuronal activation patterns in response to androgen deprivation therapy: a pilot study. BMC cancer 2010;10:1. doi: 10.1186/1471-2407-10-1

111.   Bender CM, Sereika SM, Berga SL, et al. Cognitive impairment associated with adjuvant therapy in breast cancer. Psychooncology 2006;15:422-30.

112.   Castellano JM, Kim J, Stewart FR, et al. Human apoE isoforms differentially regulate brain amyloid-beta peptide clearance. Science translational medicine 2011;3:89ra57. doi: 10.1126/scitranslmed.3002156

113.   Murphy KR, Landau SM, Choudhury KR, et al. Mapping the effects of ApoE4, age and cognitive status on 18F-florbetapir PET measured regional cortical patterns of beta-amyloid density and growth. NeuroImage 2013;78:474-80. doi: 10.1016/j.neuroimage.2013.04.048

114.   Sheline YI, Morris JC, Snyder AZ, et al. APOE4 allele disrupts resting state fMRI connectivity in the absence of amyloid plaques or decreased CSF Abeta42. J Neurosci 2010;30:17035-40. doi: 10.1523/JNEUROSCI.3987-10.2010

115.   Ponsford J, Rudzki D, Bailey K, Ng KT. Impact of apolipoprotein gene on cognitive impairment and recovery after traumatic brain injury. Neurology 2007;68:619-20.

116.   Ahles TA, Saykin AJ, Noll WW, et al. The relationship of APOE genotype to neuropsychological performance in long-term cancer survivors treated with standard dose chemotherapy. Psycho-oncology 2003;12:612-9.

117.   Small BJ, Rawson KS, Walsh E, et al. Catechol-O-methyltransferase genotype modulates cancer treatment-related cognitive deficits in breast cancer survivors. Cancer 2011;117:1369-76. doi: 10.1002/cncr.25685

118.   Caldu X, Vendrell P, Bartres-Faz D, et al. Impact of the COMT Val(108/158) Met and DAT genotypes on prefrontal function in healthy subjects. NeuroImage 2007;37:1437-44.

119.   Knight K, Wade S, Balducci L. Prevalence and outcomes of anemia in cancer: a systematic review of the literature. The American journal of medicine 2004;116 Suppl 7A:11S-26S. doi: 10.1016/j.amjmed.2003.12.008

120.   Kleinman L, Benjamin K, Viswanathan H, et al. The anemia impact measure (AIM): development and content validation of a patient-reported outcome measure of anemia symptoms and symptom impacts in cancer patients receiving chemotherapy. Quality of life research : an international journal of quality of life aspects of treatment, care and rehabilitation 2012;21:1255-66. doi: 10.1007/s11136-011-0034-1

121.   Wood SM, Meyers CA, Faderl S, Kantarjian HM, Pierce SA, Garcia-Manero G. Association of anemia and cognitive dysfunction in patients with acute myelogenous leukemia and myelodysplastic syndrome. Am J Hematol 2011;86:950-2. doi: 10.1002/ajh.22151

122.   Andro M, Le Squere P, Estivin S, Gentric A. Anaemia and cognitive performances in the elderly: a systematic review. Eur J Neurol 2013. doi: 10.1111/ene.12175

123.   Weckmann MT, Gingrich R, Mills JA, Hook L, Beglinger LJ. Risk factors for delirium in patients undergoing hematopoietic stem cell transplantation. Annals of clinical psychiatry : official journal of the American Academy of Clinical Psychiatrists 2012;24:204-14.

124.   Cruz Silva MM, Madeira VM, Almeida LM, Custodio JB. Hemolysis of human erythrocytes induced by tamoxifen is related to disruption of membrane structure. Biochimica et biophysica acta 2000;1464:49-61.

125.   Coviello AD, Kaplan B, Lakshman KM, Chen T, Singh AB, Bhasin S. Effects of graded doses of testosterone on erythropoiesis in healthy young and older men. J Clin Endocrinol Metab 2008;93:914-9. doi: 10.1210/jc.2007-1692

126.   Ahmadi H, Daneshmand S. Androgen deprivation therapy: evidence-based management of side effects. BJU international 2013;111:543-8. doi: 10.1111/j.1464-410X.2012.11774.x

127.   Stilley CS, Bender CM, Dunbar-Jacob J, Sereika S, Ryan CM. The impact of cognitive function on medication management: three studies. Health psychology 2010;29:50-5. doi: 10.1037/a0016940

128.   Hall PA, Elias LJ, Crossley M. Neurocognitive influences on health behavior in a community sample. Health Psychol 2006;25:778-82. doi: 10.1037/0278-6133.25.6.778

129.   Anderson ES, Winett RA, Wojcik JR. Self-regulation, self-efficacy, outcome expectations, and social support: social cognitive theory and nutrition behavior. Ann Behav Med 2007;34:304-12. doi: 10.1080/08836610701677659

130.   Hall PA, Fong G, Epp L, Elias LJ. Executive function moderates the intention-behavior link for physical activity and dietary behavior. Psychol & Health 2008;23:309-26.

131.   Diamond A. Biological and social influences on cognitive control processes dependent on prefrontal cortex. Progress in brain research 2011;189:319-39. doi: 10.1016/B978-0-444-53884-0.00032-4

132.   Vaishnavi SN, Vlassenko AG, Rundle MM, Snyder AZ, Mintun MA, Raichle ME. Regional aerobic glycolysis in the human brain. Proceedings of the National Academy of Sciences of the United States of America 2010;107:17757-62. doi: 10.1073/pnas.1010459107

133.   Deprez S, Billiet T, Sunaert S, Leemans A. Diffusion tensor MRI of chemotherapy-induced cognitive impairment in non-CNS cancer patients: a review. Brain Imaging Behav 2013;7:409-35. doi: 10.1007/s11682-012-9220-1

134.   Deprez S, Amant F, Yigit R, et al. Chemotherapy-induced structural changes in cerebral white matter and its correlation with impaired cognitive functioning in breast cancer patients. Human Brain Mapping 2011;32:480-93. doi: 10.1002/hbm.21033

135.   Abraham J, Haut M, Moran M, Filburn S, Lemiuex S, Kuwabara H. Adjuvant chemotherapy for breast cancer: effects on cerebral white matter seen in diffusion tensor imaging. Clin Breast Cancer 2008;8:88-91.

136.   Kohli S, Fisher SG, Tra Y, et al. The effect of modafinil on cognitive function in breast cancer survivors. Cancer 2009;115:2605-16. doi: 10.1002/cncr.24287

137. Lundorff LE, Jonsson BH, Sjogren P. Modafinil for attentional and psychomotor dysfunction in advanced cancer: a double-blind, randomised, cross-over trial. Palliative medicine 2009;23:731-8. doi: 10.1177/0269216309106872

138. Minzenberg MJ, Watrous AJ, Yoon JH, Ursu S, Carter CS. Modafinil shifts human locus coeruleus to low-tonic, high-phasic activity during functional MRI. Science 2008;322:1700-2. doi: 10.1126/science.1164908

139. Volkow ND, Fowler JS, Logan J, et al. Effects of modafinil on dopamine and dopamine transporters in the male human brain: clinical implications. JAMA 2009;301:1148-54. doi: 10.1001/jama.2009.351

140. Schwartz AL, Thompson JA, Masood N. Interferon-induced fatigue in patients with melanoma: a pilot study of exercise and methylphenidate. Oncol Nurs Forum 2002;29:E85-90. doi: 10.1188/02.ONF.E85-E90

141. Gehring K, Roukema JA, Sitskoorn MM. Review of recent studies on interventions for cognitive deficits in patients with cancer. Expert review of anticancer therapy 2012;12:255-69. doi: 10.1586/era.11.202

142. Sharma P, Wisniewski A, Braga-Basaria M, et al. Lack of an effect of high dose isoflavones in men with prostate cancer undergoing androgen deprivation therapy. J Urol 2009;182:2265-72. doi: 10.1016/j.juro.2009.07.030

143. Ferguson RJ, McDonald BC, Rocque MA, et al. Development of CBT for chemotherapy-related cognitive change: results of a waitlist control trial. Psychooncology 2012;21:176-86. doi: 10.1002/pon.1878

144. Ferguson RJ, Ahles TA, Saykin AJ, et al. Cognitive-behavioral management of chemotherapy-related cognitive change. Psychooncology 2007;16:772-7. doi: 10.1002/pon.1133

145. Gehring K, Sitskoorn MM, Gundy CM, et al. Cognitive rehabilitation in patients with gliomas: a randomized, controlled trial. J Clin Oncol 2009;27:3712-22. doi: 10.1200/JCO.2008.20.5765

146. Zucchella C, Capone A, Codella V, et al. Cognitive rehabilitation for early post-surgery inpatients affected by primary brain tumor: a randomized, controlled trial. J Neurooncol 2013. doi: 10.1007/s11060-013-1153-z

147. Hoeft F, McCandliss BD, Black JM, et al. Neural systems predicting long-term outcome in dyslexia. Proceedings of the National Academy of Sciences of the United States of America 2011;108:361-6. doi: 10.1073/pnas.1008950108

148. Turner GR, McIntosh AR, Levine B. Prefrontal Compensatory Engagement in TBI is due to Altered Functional Engagement Of Existing Networks and not Functional Reorganization. Front Syst Neurosci 2011;5:9. doi: 10.3389/fnsys.2011.00009

149. Takeuchi H, Taki Y, Sassa Y, et al. Working memory training using mental calculation impacts regional gray matter of the frontal and parietal regions. PLoS ONE 2011;6:e23175. doi: 10.1371/journal.pone.0023175

150. Takeuchi H, Taki Y, Hashizume H, et al. Effects of training of processing speed on neural systems. J Neurosci 2011;31:12139-48. doi: 10.1523/JNEUROSCI.2948-11.2011

151. Takeuchi H, Sekiguchi A, Taki Y, et al. Training of working memory impacts structural connectivity. J Neurosci 2010;30:3297-303. doi: 30/9/3297 [pii]10.1523/JNEUROSCI.4611-09.2010

152. Strangman GE, O'Neil-Pirozzi TM, Supelana C, Goldstein R, Katz DI, Glenn MB. Regional brain morphometry predicts memory rehabilitation outcome after traumatic brain injury. Frontiers in human neuroscience 2010;4:182. doi: 10.3389/fnhum.2010.00182

153. Mozolic JL, Hayasaka S, Laurienti PJ. A cognitive training intervention increases resting cerebral blood flow in healthy older adults. Front Hum Neurosci 2010;4:16. doi: 10.3389/neuro.09.016.2010

154. Klingberg T. Training and plasticity of working memory. Trends Cogn Sci 2010;14:317-24. doi: S1364-6613(10)00093-8 [pii]10.1016/j.tics.2010.05.002

155. Kim YH, Yoo WK, Ko MH, Park CH, Kim ST, Na DL. Plasticity of the attentional network after brain injury and cognitive rehabilitation. Neurorehabil Neural Repair 2009;23:468-77. doi: 1545968308328728 [pii]10.1177/1545968308328728

156. Laks J, Wolinsky FD, Vander Weg MW, Howren MB, Jones MP, Dotson MM. A Randomized Controlled Trial of Cognitive Training Using a Visual Speed of Processing Intervention in Middle Aged and Older Adults. PLoS ONE 2013;8:e61624. doi: 10.1371/journal.pone.0061624

157. Von Ah D, Carpenter JS, Saykin A, et al. Advanced cognitive training for breast cancer survivors: a randomized controlled trial. Breast Cancer Res Treat 2012;135:799-809. doi: 10.1007/s10549-012-2210-6

158. Kesler S, Hosseini SMH, Heckler C, et al. Cognitive training for improving executive function in chemotherapy-treated breast cancer survivors. Clin Breast Cancer 2013;13:299-306. doi: 10.1016/j.clbc.2013.02.004

159. Brehmer Y, Westerberg H, Backman L. Working-memory training in younger and older adults: training gains, transfer, and maintenance. Front Hum Neurosci 2012;6:63. doi: 10.3389/fnhum.2012.00063

160. Brehmer Y, Westerberg H, Bellander M, Furth D, Karlsson S, Backman L. Working memory plasticity modulated by dopamine transporter genotype. Neurosci Lett 2009;467:117-20. doi: S0304-3940(09)01328-7 [pii]10.1016/j.neulet.2009.10.018

161. Willis SL, Tennstedt SL, Marsiske M, et al. Long-term effects of cognitive training on everyday functional outcomes in older adults. JAMA 2006;296:2805-14. doi: 296/23/2805 [pii]10.1001/jama.296.23.2805

162. Haimov I, Shatil E. Cognitive Training Improves Sleep Quality and Cognitive Function among Older Adults with Insomnia. PLoS ONE 2013;8:e61390. doi: 10.1371/journal.pone.0061390

163. Riley KP, Snowdon DA, Desrosiers MF, Markesbery WR. Early life linguistic ability, late life cognitive function, and neuropathology: findings from the Nun Study. Neurobiol Aging 2005;26:341-7. doi: 10.1016/j.neurobiolaging.2004.06.019

164. Iacono D, Markesbery WR, Gross M, et al. The Nun study: clinically silent AD, neuronal hypertrophy, and linguistic skills in early life. Neurology 2009;73:665-73. doi: 10.1212/WNL.0b013e3181b01077

165. Stern Y. Cognitive reserve. Neuropsychologia 2009;47:2015-28. doi: S0028-3932(09)00123-7 [pii]10.1016/j.neuropsychologia.2009.03.004

166. Poppelreuter M, Weis J, Bartsch HH. Effects of specific neuropsychological training programs for breast cancer patients after adjuvant chemotherapy. J Psychosoc Oncol 2009;27:274-96. doi: 910064746 [pii]10.1080/07347330902776044

167. Sohlberg M, Turkstra L. Optimizing Cognitive Rehabilitation: Effective Instructional Methods. New York, NY: The Guilford Press; 2011.

168. Cicerone KD, Langenbahn DM, Braden C, et al. Evidence-based cognitive rehabilitation: updated review of the literature from 2003 through 2008. Archives of physical medicine and rehabilitation 2011;92:519-30. doi: 10.1016/j.apmr.2010.11.015

169. Toglia J, Johnston MV, Goverover Y, Dain B. A multicontext approach to promoting transfer of strategy use and self regulation after brain injury: An exploratory study. Brain Inj 2010;24:664-77. doi: 10.3109/02699051003610474

170. Von Ah D, Habermann B, Carpenter JS, Schneider BL. Impact of perceived cognitive impairment in breast cancer survivors. European journal of oncology nursing : the official journal of European Oncology Nursing Society 2013;17:236-41. doi: 10.1016/j.ejon.2012.06.002

171. Palesh O, Peppone L, Innominato PF, et al. Prevalence, putative mechanisms, and current management of sleep problems during chemotherapy for cancer. Nat Sci Sleep 2012;4:151-62. doi: 10.2147/NSS.S18895

172. Mols F, Husson O, Roukema JA, van de Poll-Franse LV. Depressive symptoms are a risk factor for all-cause mortality: results from a prospective population-based study among 3,080 cancer survivors from the PROFILES registry. J Cancer Surviv 2013. doi: 10.1007/s11764-013-0286-6

173. Esch T, Stefano GB. The neurobiology of stress management. Neuro Endocrinol Lett 2010;31:19-39.

174. Rubia K. The neurobiology of Meditation and its clinical effectiveness in psychiatric disorders. Biol Psychol 2009;82:1-11. doi: 10.1016/j.biopsycho.2009.04.003

175. Moran A, Guillot A, Macintyre T, Collet C. Re-imagining motor imagery: building bridges between cognitive neuroscience and sport psychology. Br J Psychol 2012;103:224-47. doi: 10.1111/j.2044-8295.2011.02068.x

176. Langdon KD, Corbett D. Improved working memory following novel combinations of physical and cognitive activity. Neurorehabil Neural Repair 2012;26:523-32. doi: 10.1177/1545968311425919

177. Denkinger MD, Nikolaus T, Denkinger C, Lukas A. Physical activity for the prevention of cognitive decline : Current evidence from observational and controlled studies. Zeitschrift fur Gerontologie und Geriatrie 2012;45:11-6. doi: 10.1007/s00391-011-0262-6

178. Ahlskog JE, Geda YE, Graff-Radford NR, Petersen RC. Physical exercise as a preventive or disease-modifying treatment of dementia and brain aging. Mayo Clinic proceedings Mayo Clinic 2011;86:876-84. doi: 10.4065/mcp.2011.0252

179.   Janelsins M, Peppone L, Heckler C, et al. YOCAS yoga, fatigue, memory difficulty, and quality of life: Results from a URCC CCOP randomized, controlled clinical trial among 358 cancer survivors. J Clin Oncol 2012;30:abstr 9142.

180.   Mustian K, Palesh OG, Sprod L, et al. Effect of YOCAS yoga on sleep, fatigue, and quality of life: A URCC CCOP randomized, controlled clinical trial among 410 cancer survivors. J Clin Oncol 2010;28:abstr 9013.

181.   Mustian K, Sprod L, Peppone L, et al. Effect of YOCAS yoga on circadian rhythm, anxiety, and mood: A URCC CCOP randomized, controlled clinical trial among 410 cancer survivors. J Clin Oncol 2011;29:abstr 9034.

182.   Sprod LK, Mohile SG, Demark-Wahnefried W, et al. Exercise and Cancer Treatment Symptoms in 408 Newly Diagnosed Older Cancer Patients. Journal of geriatric oncology 2012;3:90-7. doi: 10.1016/j.jgo.2012.01.002

183.   Curlik DM, 2nd, Shors TJ. Training your brain: Do mental and physical (MAP) training enhance cognition through the process of neurogenesis in the hippocampus? Neuropharmacology 2013;64:506-14. doi: 10.1016/j.neuropharm.2012.07.027

184.   Kramer AF, Erickson KI, Colcombe SJ. Exercise, cognition, and the aging brain. Journal of Applied Physiology 2006;101:1237-42. doi: 10.1152/japplphysiol.00500.2006

185.   Speisman RB, Kumar A, Rani A, Foster TC, Ormerod BK. Daily exercise improves memory, stimulates hippocampal neurogenesis and modulates immune and neuroimmune cytokines in aging rats. Brain Behav Immun 2013;28:25-43. doi: 10.1016/j.bbi.2012.09.013

186.   Pietrelli A, Lopez-Costa J, Goni R, Brusco A, Basso N. Aerobic exercise prevents age-dependent cognitive decline and reduces anxiety-related behaviors in middle-aged and old rats. Neuroscience 2012;202:252-66. doi: 10.1016/j.neuroscience.2011.11.054

187.   Rock CL, Byers TE, Colditz GA, et al. Reducing breast cancer recurrence with weight loss, a vanguard trial: the Exercise and Nutrition to Enhance Recovery and Good Health for You (ENERGY) Trial. Contemporary clinical trials 2013;34:282-95. doi: 10.1016/j.cct.2012.12.003

188.   Burke LE, Conroy MB, Sereika SM, et al. The effect of electronic self-monitoring on weight loss and dietary intake: a randomized behavioral weight loss trial. Obesity (Silver Spring) 2011;19:338-44. doi: 10.1038/oby.2010.208

189.   Acharya SD, Elci OU, Sereika SM, Styn MA, Burke LE. Using a personal digital assistant for self-monitoring influences diet quality in comparison to a standard paper record among overweight/obese adults. J Am Diet Assoc 2011;111:583-8. doi: 10.1016/j.jada.2011.01.009

190.   Burke LE, Styn MA, Sereika SM, et al. Using mHealth technology to enhance self-monitoring for weight loss: a randomized trial. Am J Prev Med 2012;43:20-6. doi: 10.1016/j.amepre.2012.03.016

191.   Burke LE, Wang J, Sevick MA. Self-monitoring in weight loss: a systematic review of the literature. J Am Diet Assoc 2011;111:92-102. doi: 10.1016/j.jada.2010.10.008

192.   Brunet J, Taran S, Burke S, Sabiston CM. A qualitative exploration of barriers and motivators to physical activity participation in women treated for breast cancer. Disabil Rehabil 2013. doi: 10.3109/09638288.2013.802378